MINDFULNESS IN EVERYDAY LIFE

Techniques on how to set your mind and body for dealing with anxiety, stress, and personal loss. How to improve mental health.

Collection of Five Yoga and Mindfulness Meditation Books for Beginners

by George M. Posi

Books in Collection "MINDFULNESS IN EVERYDAY LIFE"

MINDFULNESS YOGA AND MEDITATION

PROCRASTINATION: HOW TO STOP WASTING
YOUR TIME

MINDFULNESS: THE BENEFITS OF MEDITATION

USE MINDFULNESS MEDITATION TO STOP
PROCRASTINATING

A BEGINNER'S GUIDE TO YOGA MEDITATION

INTRODUCTION

I want to thank you and congratulate you on reading the book "Mindfulness in everyday life." This book contains proven steps and strategies for how to relieve stress, find happiness in your life, create your inner peace, and make your experience better.

Mindfulness meditation will help you to remain calm and in the present moment. You will learn to live in this moment. You do not have control over your past or your future. Mindfulness meditation teaches you the importance of what you are doing now and space through which you are moving at each moment.

Bottom line: mindfulness is the practice of focusing all your attention on the present moment purposefully and accepting it resolutely without judgment. It's a perfect place to begin if you are looking for true peace and happiness.

Meditative techniques are an essential part of any yoga exercise. Even though you don't need to formally meditate to practice yoga, the two practices support each other. Through your practice of yoga, you enhance both your ability to concentrate and to relax. Those are the two most essential requirements for meditation practice. Here, you can deepen your understanding of what meditation is and begin a practice of your own.

Thanks again for reading this book. I hope you enjoy it!

Mindfulness

YOGA AND MEDITATION, SIMPLE BEGINNERS GUIDE TO STRESS RELIEF AND HAPPINESS

Techniques on how to set your mind and body for dealing with anxiety, stress and personal loss. How to improve your mental health trough wisdom of Buddhism, Zen and other spiritual practices, create your inner peace and make your life better

GEORGE M. POSI

BOOK 1: MINDFULNESS YOGA AND MEDITATION

Simple Beginners Guide To Stress Relief And Happiness

Table of contents

THE STRESS AND ANXIETY PROBLEM IN PERSPECTIVE

A s I mentioned earlier, I know you're here today because stress and anxiety have taken its toll on you, and from what you've been experiencing, you can already tell that it's on course to make things worse in your life.

Regardless of what the source of your stress is, you might already be feeling hopeless and miserable because you cannot live life normally. You may not be happy or productive at your place of work, you are always making enemies and you probably even have to deal with some emotional and mental issues such as anxiety, panic attacks and phobias that are driving you crazy.

I understand that when you are stressed, it can be tough for you to focus, make sound decisions, and properly think things through or even recall the simplest things. The stress may contribute to extreme irritability, which makes you easily impatient with other people and frustrated and, at times, yet causing depression, feelings of insecurity, anger, and conflicts in your relationships.

The physical effects of stress can also be very overwhelming; you might even be experiencing muscle tension, which is one of the most common physical reactions to stress. I know that to a certain level, stress can trigger tension headaches and even migraines, among other musculoskeletal conditions. By extension, your digestive system could also be suffering under the effects of stress, particularly considering that stress affects the nutrients being absorbed by the intestines.

It also influences the speed of the food movement through your body, which means that you may already be eating less or more than you would typically do. Moreover, I know that this disruption of the natural digestive processes of your body can lead to pain, vomiting, constipation, diarrhea, acid reflux, nausea, and heartburn. One or two of these issues can easily make your life utterly unbearable.

In other words, what you're going through is already damaging and can get worse if you don't do anything about it; even worse, ignoring or trying to acclimate yourself to these effects can only make things a lot worse.

Before we talk about the stress management techniques, let me give you a bit of insight into what goes on in your body when stressed.

What happens when stress strikes?

When you are stressed, there are physical and chemical changes your brain undergoes, which affects its normal functioning. When your stress levels are high, the body releases stress hormones like cortisol.

Cortisol does several things in your body, such as increasing your blood pressure and heart rate, and your immune system becomes weak because your body is concentrating on what is essential, and that is to "fight or flee" the stressor.

If you don't make an effort to control the stress, it may become chronic and cause a host of other problems such as stroke, ulcers, heart disease, and asthma. Besides, you need to note that a good number of health care experts actually link chronic stress with many deadly illnesses such as heart attacks and cancer.

Among the reasons is that the reaction of your body to prolonged stress can build up slowly as you try to 'get used to' constant pressure. Nonetheless, even when you seem to be successfully creating some level of tolerance to stress, your nervous system continues to deal with an overflow in the background which can, in the long run, have a grave impact on your overall health, causing some of the mental and physical issues we discussed earlier.

So, what can you do to make a shift into a healthier pattern, reduce stress, and be happier? Practice mindfulness meditation and yoga. They are simple yet one of the most effective techniques we have today.

Let us learn more about mindfulness meditation and yoga in the next chapter.

WHAT IS MINDFULNESS MEDITATION AND YOGA

L et us start by understanding mindfulness meditation, and then we can move on to Yoga.

Mindfulness Meditation

Mindfulness meditation is a powerful ancient technique that has been used for years, mainly to reduce stress, anxiety, depression, and achieve inner peace. It has also been used to relieve pain and treat certain illnesses. But what exactly is mindfulness meditation?

Mindfulness meditation re-trains your mind to remain in the 'now' or present moment, entirely calm as it should be. Many times, we become anxious and stressed because of a disturbing past that we keep thinking about or worrying about a future that you have no control over. With mindfulness meditation, you learn to live in the moment only, as that is what you can change as you have no control over your past or future.

While its exact origin is still somewhat vague, the practices and instructions of mindfulness meditation have been found in the ancient texts of many major religions such as Judaism, Buddhism, and Hinduism. Even so, Buddhism plays a pivotal role in helping us understand the concept of mindfulness meditation; the practice is integral to the 'Buddhist path.' In Buddhism, cultivating non-judgmental awareness of yourself, your feelings, and your mind is considered very important.

You need to understand that this practice suggests that it is essential for the mind to fully attend to what is taking place, to what you are doing, and to space through which you are moving. Every so often, we veer from the issue at hand; our mind takes flight, we stop being in touch with our body and slowly become absorbed in obsessive thoughts about stuff that has already taken place or continuously worry about the future. That creates anxiety. Yet, regardless of how far away we drift, mindfulness is there to take us back to where we are and what we are feeling and doing.

Bottom-line: mindfulness in itself is, therefore, the practice of focusing all your attention on the present moment purposefully and accepting it resolutely without judgment. It's a perfect place to begin if you are looking for true peace and happiness.

Yoga

Yoga is another ancient practice that is highly regarded as one of the most effective ways to manage stress, cultivate happiness, and peace of mind in addition to reducing body pain, increasing flexibility and body strength. There are many ways to define or look at this restorative practice, though- here are some of them:

Yoga is a 'connection' or 'union.' In Sanskrit, the word is usually used to denote *connection*. Yoga can thus be defined as *the state of a connection* or a set of techniques that let you connect to anything (see the next chapter to have a better understanding).

Looking at it at the most practical level, you will find that yoga is the whole process of being more aware of who you are. Its techniques bring about health and balance and are meant to unfold your dormant, hidden potential. Yoga allows you to be more aware of yourself and feels more connected. This makes the practice a process of self-discovery, which guides you to self-realization and self-mastery.

But where did it originate from?

The origin of yoga is also not very clear, but researchers think the practice is about 10,000 years old. However, its development can be traced back to more than 5,000 years ago. Some experts maintain that Northern India was the place where Yoga began by what is known as the "Indus-Sarasvati" civilization. The first mention of the word 'yoga' is noted in the oldest sacred texts known as the Rig Veda. The Vedas were set of documents that contained mantras, texts, rituals, and songs, which were used by the Vedic priests, who were referred to as the Brahmans.

Bottom-line:

When done right, yoga and mindfulness will reduce the amount of time you usually spend feeling overwhelmed and help you appreciate every little moment as it comes. In a chaotic world, spiritual practices like yoga and mindfulness might be all you would need to learn so that you can cope with all the madness.

Before we move on to how to practice mindfulness meditation and yoga, let us first learn how exactly these two practices enable you to deal with stress better:

How Yoga And Mindfulness Meditation Do The Magic (A Brief Annotation)

Mind-body therapies like yoga and meditation are becoming more popular every day in the field of mental health for promoting psychological well-being. That makes a lot of sense because science has proven countless times that mindfulness skills can actually help with anxiety and improve mood.

To start with, yoga helps with depression by working with your tendency to dwell on certain feelings, thoughts, or emotions and dysfunctional thought patterns. A simple yoga session can help you notice the shifts in mood and guide you to learn coping strategies that encourage you to practice observing instead of judging such changes in attitude. If you have the tendency to have negative thought patterns, these skills can help you counteract that, and in the process, help you improve issues of depression.

The physical aspect of yoga is also essential and effective in counteracting the agitation and inactivity that usually comes with anxiety and depression. This means that you get to be more active and less agitated by people or things around you. This works as you develop a sense of self-mastery, which is a very crucial part that you need if you are to manage stress effectively.

For instance, when you are doing yoga or meditation, a sense of accomplishment and self-mastery is instilled as you learn to maintain a connection with your breath as (in the case of yoga) you hold or transition through the poses, despite the potential distractions like losing focus or balance.

Finally, a regular meditation and yoga practice can cultivate in you a sense of active participation in working through your issues and having a sense of control over yourself as regards to the improvement in your emotional well-being; you get to understand that 'you are the one in control of your emotional progress and happiness.'

HOW TO PRACTICE YOGA: GETTING STARTED

P reparation is vital in the whole practice of yoga and meditation. It determines the success or failure of the practice. So, what are you supposed to do here?

Dedicate some space and time

The place you choose for your practice has to be calm, quiet, and soothing. You also want to pick a convenient time, which you are unlikely to be interrupted. If possible, you can create some space in your house that is rarely used. It should be peaceful and one that can encourage you to relax as you practice mindfulness and yoga. You should not use this space to do anything else apart from these spiritual practices. That way, when you sit down, your mind and body will instantly switch to calmness and be ready to begin the practice effortlessly.

Ground yourself

You also have to ground yourself, especially just before you start your session. Grounding is a term that refers to calming your mind and being consciously aware of the present moment. It is generally divided into two categories:
- Connecting yourself with your body
- Attaching yourself to the earth, particularly before meditating (this means being aware of the force of gravity on your body- think of it as being literally grounded)

What to do to connect with the earth each time you are on the mat, ready to begin meditating:

Notice any imbalance of your body weight either front to back or left to right and try to correct that imbalance; if your body is tilted in one direction, you will feel like you are falling over.

After that, release any stiffness in your muscles to allow your body tissues to be soft and fold to the surface below them. Smooth muscles are critical as they create a fuller base and bring the feeling of "being planted."

Next, make you are sitting upright, comfortable, and relaxed by releasing your psoas. This instruction is mostly used in yoga sessions. In meditation or yoga, the psoas is referred to as the deep muscle in the core that connects your torso to each leg.

Confused? Think of it this way; the psoas is the region deep in your core that tends to become tight sometimes and typically brings about the 'gripping' feeling- you know, as though you need to hold or brace yourself upright. When you release your psoas, sitting tends to feel a lot easier, and it gives the feeling that the earth is supporting you and not your muscles.

Lastly, imagine roots growing deep down into the earth. At that moment, visualizing that creates some energetic connection with the earth.

What to do to connect to your body (or becoming embodied for a better yoga and mindfulness meditation experience)

When you dwell on your thoughts, you will rarely be in the present moment. The good thing is that your body always lives in the present moment, and that makes it different. It can only experience sensations that are taking place at this moment, even as your mind is lost in the past or future. Therefore, being able to be aware of your body means being able to connect with the present. When it comes to the nervous system, this is very soothing. It calms the mind and makes it easier to meditate. This is what you need to do to connect with your body:

- Have a conscious awareness of your feet, back, and pelvis
- Be aware of your body sensations
- Be mindful of your breath.

When you ground yourself, sitting upright becomes more comfortable, your nervous system becomes calm, and you are generally able to come to and remain in the present moment, which are the main ingredients in making your meditation a lot easier.

In summary (or in case you got lost somewhere) grounding yourself asks the following of you:

- Bring some awareness to the lower part of your body- that is, your feet or pelvis, and then to the back of your body.
- Pay attention to your inhalation and exhalation.
- Gently notice the support sensations below the body- that is, the cushion, chair, or ground.
- Notice your body sensations, which include what you are hearing, smelling, tasting, seeing, or feeling.
- Imagine the roots growing from your body's base into the earth.
- Feel the energy spiraling down your spine, and into the earth's core.
- Bring awareness to your body's heaviness (at the base) and then feel the lift of your spine upward.

Note:

In any practice of mindfulness and yoga, it is always essential to have tools that make it simpler. When you plop yourself on the cushion, it simply means that you might struggle to start meditating, and if you've already begun, you may have a problem continuing. When you, however, take a moment to ground yourself and prepare yourself for the practice, your mind and body become primed. You thus struggle a lot less, and your practice goes on smoothly.

Create Contentment

Just before you start meditating, it is crucial to create contentment in your body as much as you can. Ideally, you should make your bodily comfort a priority before you start your practice. You should also do what you can to avoid starting the session too full or too hungry, for instance. Also, try to wear clothing that is easy on your body and put any electronic devices away. If possible, switch them off altogether because you want as few distractions as possible that separate you from the practice. Take a couple of moments before you start setting an intention for the practice. This could be something as simple as 'ease my anxiety' or 'stay present.' It doesn't matter what your aim is- you can go back to it in your practice to keep yourself on track.

And finally, practice a starter pose!

Sometimes all you need to get prepared for a good meditation session—whether in the form of mindfulness meditation or yoga is a right yoga pose or a few mindful yoga poses. In this case, paying attention to your breathing and doing your best to be wholly absorbed by your practice is the key to success. The yoga practice you select should be able to assist you to loosen up your body and be able to work out whatever kinks that could potentially bring about discomfort in your meditation. You will also have a clear mind so that you don't have many distracting thoughts floating in your brain when the time to sit or start your main movements comes.

While you can choose a starter pose that you like, this one always does the trick:

The Mountain Pose

This pose develops physical and mental strength, which is essential when you are particularly feeling overwhelmed by stress or anxiety. It is referred to as the mother of all asanas (poses) because the other asanas emerge from it.

How to do it

1. Stand in an erect position, legs slightly apart, and your hands hanging beside your body.
2. Try to firm your thigh muscles and lift your kneecaps, making sure that you don't harden the lower section of your stomach.
3. Now try to strengthen your inner ankles' inner arches while lifting them.
4. Visualize a stream of energy (in the form of white light) passing through your ankles, all the way to your inner thighs, spine, neck, and head. Turn your upper legs inward gently and then elongate your tailbone toward the floor. Now raise the pubis towards the navel.
5. Look upward slightly and then breathe in. As you do so, stretch your arms, shoulders, and chest towards the sky. Slowly raise your heels and make sure your body weight is resting on your toes.
6. Feel your body stretch from your feet all the way to your head. Hold the pose for a couple of seconds, and then breathe out, and come out of the pose.

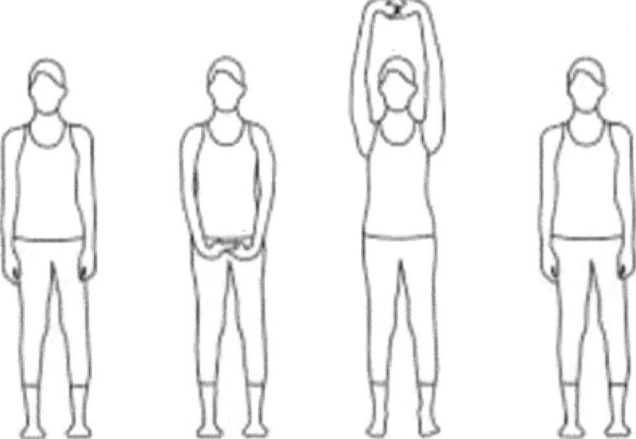

The following chapter will focus on more yoga poses for stress relief.

YOGA POSES FOR STRESS RELIEF

L et us now learn some yoga poses you can do to release stress;

Cat Pose to Cow Pose

The cat pose is one that gives your spine as well as the belly organs a gentle massage and acts as an excellent stress buster. Usually, this pose is paired with the cow pose (at the point of inhalation) to offer the best overall health benefits, which include better stimulation of the digestive tract and spinal fluid. The cow pose is a straightforward and gentle way to get your spine warmed up. Besides relieving stress and tension and calming the mind, the pose also helps in creating emotional balance.

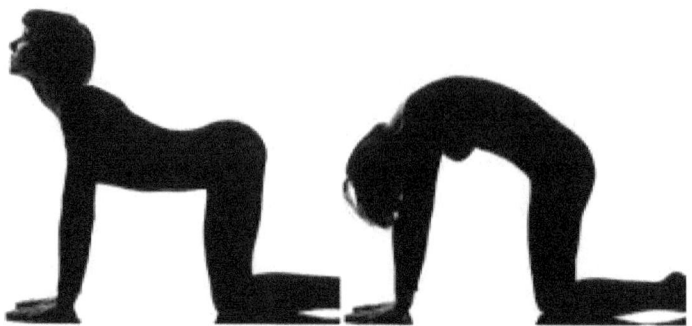

How to do it

1. Start by placing your knees and hands on the floor. Ensure the knees are below your hips, and the wrists are firmly placed beneath the shoulders. Have your spine in a neutral position; your back should be flat and abs engaged. Breathe in deeply.

2. As you breathe out, assume the cow pose by rounding your spine upwards. Imagine yourself pulling your navel up towards your spine as you engage your abs. Bring your chin back toward your chest, tuck it in and then release your neck to form the cat-like shape.

3. As you breathe in, arch your back and then relax your belly. Raise your head and tailbone upwards. Don't place any unnecessary stress on your neck.

4. Keep flowing from the cat pose to the cow pose back and forth and connect your breath to the movements. Repeat the steps for a minimum of 10 rounds or until your spine warms up.

The Child's Pose

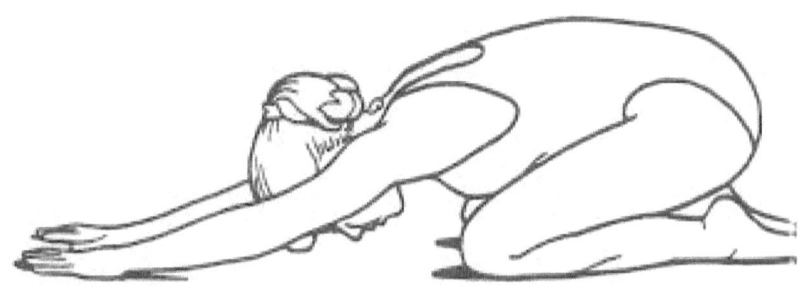

This is one of those few yoga poses that allow you to rest your forehead on the ground, which has been seen to really help in relieving anxiety. Indeed, it is a restful pose that you can sequence between the poses you find more challenging. You can also do this pose with your arms alongside your body as opposed to having them over your head.

How to do it

1. Place your sit-bones over your heels and stretch out your hands in front of you. Fold your torso forward slowly until the center of your eyebrow rests on the mat.
2. Let your big toes touch and place your knees together or just let them stay separate but wider than the hips.
3. While you can stack your forearms and hands and rest your head there, traditionally, you are supposed to rest the arms back alongside your body, with palms facing up.
4. In case your butt or hips don't touch the heels, you can also put a cushion in between so that you can relax and let go. Stay like that for 10 or so breaths, letting go as much as you can each time you breathe out.

Standing Forward Fold

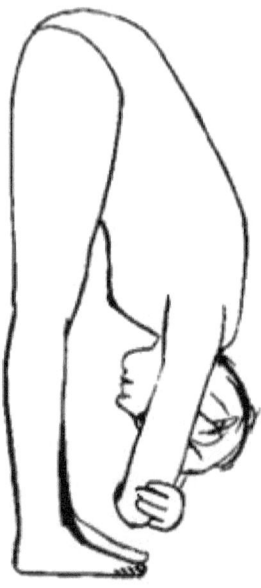

This pose is one of the best when it comes to balancing the nervous system, quieting your mind, and promoting peace and calmness. It balances and calms down excessive and fluctuating emotional energy by adjusting what is known as the 'sacral chakra.'

How to do it

1. The first step to this pose should be the mountain pose (see above).
2. After completing the mountain pose, bend your knees and engage your core slightly, while hinging forward from your hips and place your hands in front of your feet or alongside (beside) them.
3. Shift your weight onto the padded region of your feet (balls of your feet) and then feel your sit bones lifting upwards. You can continue bending your knees to tighten your hamstrings and protect your lower back.
4. You can, however, try lengthening through the back of your legs as you keep the weight on your padded feet regions.
5. Hold each one of your elbows with the opposite hand and soften around your head, neck, jaw, eyes, and mind.
6. Hold the position for a couple of breaths and then come out of the pose very slowly.

Reclined Angle Pose

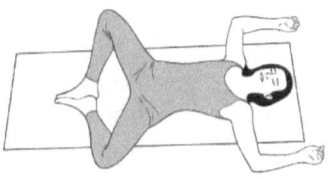

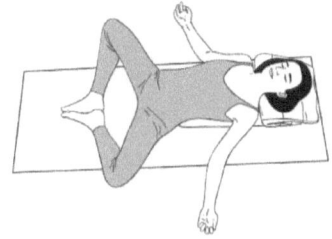

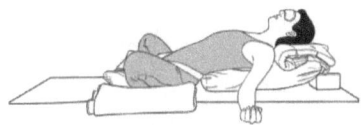

This pose gives you that feeling that you are taking a mini-vacation. The posture can assist you open through your groin, inner thighs, and hips, among other places that stress and tension might be hiding. With the floor beneath you, supporting you fully, you can surrender yourself to the moment and let go.

How to do it

1. Lie on your back as the pictures above illustrate and then bring together the soles of your feet, with knees out to the sides. If you find your knees significantly far from the floor, use some yoga blocks, folded blankets or bolsters and place them beneath your knees to increase the restorative power of the pose.

2. There are many ways you can position your arms. For one, you can raise them overhead and grab each elbow with the opposite hand, or rest them on the floor beside your torso. Alternatively, you can place your right hand on the heart

center, and the other one on your belly to create a calming connection within yourself.

3. Remain in that position for a period that feels comfortable, and then come out of the pose slowly when you are ready to do so.

Remember: This pose offers a great chance to reinforce a calming, positive message to yourself. You can repeat such words as, "I am letting go," or "I am relaxed and calm."

The Plow Pose

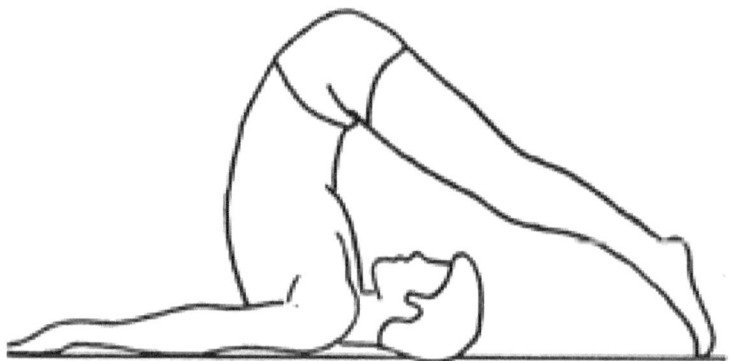

The plow pose is another fantastic stress-buster that improves blood flow to the brain, releases the head, neck, shoulders all the way to the hamstrings. The pose also helps you breathe and turns you inward.

I love this pose due to the way it calms my brain and reduces fatigue by giving my spine and shoulders a perfect stretch. If you also want to enjoy these and more benefits:

Do the following

1. Lie on your back, and rest your arms beside your body, with palms facing downwards.
2. Breathe in and lift your feet off the ground with your abdominal muscles. Let your legs be at an angle of 90 degrees.
3. Support your hips using your hands and lift them off the floor; place your feet at an angle of 180 degrees, in such a way that your toes go over and beyond your head. If you are not that flexible, you can just take them as far back as you can.
4. Ensure your back is perpendicular to the floor

5.   Hold the pose for a minute as you focus on your breath. Breathe out and bring your legs down gently. Try not to jerk your legs as you release the pose.

Note: As a beginner, you run the risk of overstretching your neck when you do this pose. Your goal is to be pushing down the tops of your shoulders to have your shoulders lifted a bit towards your ear and back well supported. This makes sure the rear of your neck and throat are soft. Also, press your shoulder blades against your back firmly to open your sternum up.

You can perform these yoga poses in a series once you select the ones you like or after arranging them in order, you think works best for you. You can also combine them with mindfulness meditation. Let us learn how to actually practice mindfulness meditation.

HOW TO PRACTICE MINDFULNESS MEDITATION

B efore we begin, you need to realize that there is no perfect way to do mindfulness meditation. Different people have different methods or forms of doing mindfulness practices. Some people do it in the form of a prayer, some infuse it with yoga meditation, and others build their practice around different accouterments such as incense and candles- and sit for hours on end gazing.

You will find many different mindfulness meditation variations and techniques all over the place, but all you need is a straightforward intention, the simple method, and a tiny bit of time.

That said, follow the below steps to practice mindfulness meditation:

Find a comfortable sitting position

You can just begin by sitting on the floor cross-legged or in a chair. Straighten out your back and neck and put your hand in your lap. Look down about three or so feet in front of you.

Close your eyes

If you don't feel like closing your eyes, it's also okay to keep them open-especially if you are comfortable gazing at a steady point away from you or at the floor (this is necessary to create focus).

You can also let your eyelids fall naturally so that they stay about half open, keeping in mind that you are more likely to fall asleep if you keep your eyes closed as you meditate (which can be a problem). On the other hand, trying to keep your eyes half-open may feel odd at first and distract you. For now, whatever feels right and effortless is ideal.

Focus

Hold it for a moment. Before we continue, you need to keep a few things in mind:

Different types of meditation prescribe different ways of focusing your attention. Some of them include the following:

- Focusing on the breath
- Focusing on a mantra
- Focusing on your steps
- Focusing on your thoughts

This book is the first in upcoming series on how to manage stress, cultivate happiness, and peace of mind. Forthcoming publications will go more in-depth on topics described in this book, including different types of meditation in various Buddhist traditions.

Focus on the breath

Among the purest forms of meditating is focusing on your breath. You need to pay attention as you breathe in and breathe out. As we are going to see shortly, mindfulness meditation does not require you to breathe in any particular way but breathe as you would normally, but paying attention to it. If your mind wanders, bring it back to your breath.

In mindfulness meditation, you are basically concentrating on something very lightly and loosely as you become mindful of all that arises within your range of awareness (such as being clearly aware in an all-inclusive and open way). While that sounds nice when you are just starting out, it might not be the prettiest. This is how it looks:

...you focus on your breath, then four seconds later, you lose concentration, you wake up three minutes later (and take a few seconds to ask yourself what happened). You return to your breath and then lose focus, wake up two minutes later (maybe curse a bit), and go back to your breath...

As you start, know that this is very normal and appreciate the fact that your mind, with time, will begin quieting and becoming evident.

Lastly, you need to note that you can focus in any form (not just sitting down), which includes standing anywhere, such as in your living room, outside, or in your office, even for a couple of seconds. This means there are no restrictions to the practice, yet though it is usually done as a form of sitting meditation for a couple of minutes at a time. You can sit down and meditate as short as 10 minutes and up to an hour.

That said, let's continue (with the steps).

Turn your attention to the process of breathing. You now need to follow each inhalation and exhalation from start to finish, firmly but softly. As I mentioned, you should not try to control your breath here but observe it silently. This silent observation will slowly and gently start calming your breathing naturally. While this is easier said than done, particularly in the beginning, you still have to make an effort.

Count every inhale and exhale

This is simple. You breathing in... and count one, breathing out... and count two. Continue counting until you reach ten. If you are distracted by a thought, start the count over, starting from one. When you get to ten successfully, thank yourself and start over and try counting to ten once more. Don't worry if you never reach ten. You know that with time, you will.

You can take days or weeks; just try to achieve that goal (of counting to ten with very little or no effort) regardless of the amount of time it takes.

After that, count each inhalation and exhalation as one. When it becomes smooth and completely effortless, then stop counting and just follow your breath. Progress as slowly as you can.

Acknowledge your feelings, thoughts and any sensation that arises

You have to understand beforehand that while being mindful, you'll get various emotions, thoughts, and sensations, which may make you lose your concentration on your breath. As you are just getting started, you are likely to be interrupted every now and then and feel as though you are not doing it right. Understand that staying concentrated on the breath is not easy for anyone, particularly when they are just getting started.

Go back to being mindful of your breath

As I said, be prepared to lose focus on your breathing several times at first. Just remain focused, and after a short while, your mind will start growing quieter.

Don't forget that the practice will get better usually in a brief period – in just a couple of weeks, you should begin noticing a remarkably calm and tranquil mind.

Focus on a mantra

Another great way to practice mindfulness meditation is by using a mantra. A mantra is a syllable, phrase, or word that you repeat during meditation. You can whisper, speak, chant, or repeat the mantra in your mind. For instance, 'Aum' or 'Om' is a popular sound people repeatedly use as a mantra.

You may be wondering, is mantra meditation effective? Well, it is. As meditation gurus will tell you, a mantra employs the thinking mind and "uses thoughts to go beyond thoughts."

In Buddhism traditions, mantra chanting has a sacred meaning and has been widely practiced for ages. For instance, in Mahayana Buddhism, mantras are deeply chanted related to the different forms of the Buddha. The practice is also practiced in many other Buddhist traditions.

I could go on and on about how widespread and deep the practice of mantra is to the Buddhists, but hopefully, you get the point. Mantra meditation is regarded as one of those techniques that stop subtle and compulsive thinking; by repeating it slowly, it gradually makes it (the mantra) quieten down to a whisper in the mind until it finally stops.

In this state (when you do it right), you can be able to create profound changes in your psyche and body and produce altered states of consciousness which help you to be calm, peaceful and blissful.

But how do you pick your mantra?

- One of the things you have to do is be aware of the meaning of the words you are thinking of using as your mantra. You have to select a word that represents something you really want to develop in yourself, connect to, or feel more. It could be freedom, love, courage, peace, awareness, light, and so forth.

- Secondly, the sound of the word has to "speak" to you. To get the sound that works for you most, you have to repeat it a few minutes and observe how it makes you feel before and after.

When you decide on the mantra that works for you best, focus on using that one mantra so that its effects genuinely build you up.

The more you repeat your mantra, the more it becomes magnetized or energized in you. After some time, it will get a life of its own owing to the repeated attention you give it. It becomes the most influential thought in your mind that you can rely on for calmness and peace.

Finally, as your mantra gains momentum, repeating it becomes increasingly effortless to such an extent that you just 'log into' or 'start,' and it goes on by itself, taking you into inner silence.

That said, this is what you should do when you decide what mantra you want to use:

- You can start by repeating your mantra aloud. This will engage more of your senses and make it simpler to focus.

- Then, you can whisper the mantra (the tongue and lips move) so that there is no audible sound coming. This is deeper and subtler than the verbal recitation.

- After some time, try reciting and repeating it in your mind. When you are just starting, you will have some natural movement in your tongue and throat, but with time, the action will all cease, and the practice becomes completely mental.

- Next, you want to synchronize the mantra with the rhythm of your breathing. If your mantra is short like 'love,' you can repeat it once as you breathe in and once more when breathing out. You can also increase its speed and repeat it twice or thrice when breathing in and the same count when breathing out. The number of times you go over in one breath should depend on how you feel.

Soon, you will reach a level known as casual listening, where you are no longer repeating the mantra. The word is instead going on in your mind by itself spontaneously, all the time. At this point, you don't have to worry about its speed, loudness, and so forth. All you have to do is listen to it being repeated when it naturally wants to be repeated. This level is also known as Ajapa Japa.

Focusing on your steps

You can also meditate outside your house while walking. This is walking without a particular destination or goal (at least without focusing on either of them). You instead are aware and focus on each step as well as your breath. Basics are the same as described in meditation focused on breathing. Just pay attention to your body and gently direct thoughts back to it when they begin straying.

- Practice walking meditation wearing shoes or preferably barefoot.
- It is vital to choose a place where you file safe and with fewer distractions as possible. Set a straight path of about 10 to 15 meters (30-40 feet) long, and stand upright, with eyes pointed down at about 45 degrees.
- Take a few deep breaths and star walking at some slower pace.
- Set your attention at the soles of the feet, on the sensations as they arise and pass away.
- Feel every sensation in your feet, and movement of the legs as they swing through the air.
- As you become aware of the movement of the foot, you should note two parts of the step: lifting parts and dropping elements.
- As you lift the foot, repeat to your self "lifting." When you put it down, then say to your self "dropping."
- After some time, making your step slower so that you can easily note the movement of the foot.
- As you master how to note lifting and dropping, then you can notice the next object. Three parts of a step must be acknowledged: lifting, pushing, and dropping part. When you lift the foot, recognize lifting. When you push it forward, you just accept "pushing." When you drop it down, you will acknowledge "dropping."
- Walk back and forth along the same path. When you come to the end of your path, come to a full stop, turn around, stop again, and then start again.
- From time to time, ask yourself where your mind is now. If it is not on the soles of the feet, gently bring it back and reestablish mindfulness.
- Walk at least 15 minutes, but no more than one hour.

When you develop the ability to focus while walking like this, you will also be able to integrate it in walks in your everyday life.

Focusing on your thoughts

Mindfulness meditation is a technique that allows observing your own thoughts as they come, without judging them or getting too caught up in them. All you have to do is mindfully note them and allow them to pass. In Buddhism, this technique is also known as Vipassana. Instead of focusing only on your breath, you focus on every sensation, thought, or action you take. The process of Vipassana meditation is similar to meditation focusing on breathing, but, while you are focusing on your breath, you stay open to all sensations that may arrive. With consistent practice, you will find out that the content of your mind does not matter. What matters is how you let it affect you. You will learn that instead of getting lost in your thoughts, you can choose to watch them come and go. They can only hold power over you if you blindly follow them wherever they lead.

So, how to perform meditation focused on your thoughts?

- Sit and relax as in meditation, focused on the breath. Actually, you will start your meditation as you are going to be focused on your breathing.

- Now, you note arriving sensations or thoughts, let them go and move on. If you try to fight them, they will prevail.

- When you hear a sound, you say to yourself: "Sound, sound, sound." When you think about someone or something, you just acknowledge that and say: "Thought, thought, thought." If you are cold, say: "cold, cold, cold."

- You just accept that your mind is wandering around and want to be occupied with sensations happening around you, or some good or bad things in your life, much more than to be in a present moment.

- Do not let those thoughts take over your mind, just calmly acknowledge them, and gently bring back focus to your breath.

Vipassana meditation is one of the more sophisticated techniques and requires experienced practitioners of mindful meditation. You start with a meditation focused on your breath, followed by some walking meditation or mantra, and slowly progress to this higher form, but in time you will be able to it better and better.

The next step will be to introduce mindfulness into your daily routine and be aware of every moment as it happens.

Remember

As you start the practice, you will notice that thoughts will intrude on your silence, but with time, you will be able to quieten all the thinking long enough so that all is left is some kind of joyful and peaceful emptiness of awareness.

All you have to remember is that when thoughts inevitably rise as you recite your mantra, gently try to keep in touch with the vast silence that's always waiting for you in the background.

As I mentioned before, you can practice yoga and mindfulness together for better results once you've understood the fundamentals of both practices. Your goal can be to do a pose like the "child's" pose while focusing on your breath or chanting your mantra for a more relaxed and blissful experience.

PROCRASTINATION

HOW TO STOP WASTING YOUR TIME AND BE MORE PRODUCTIVE

Simple guide how to cure laziness, set goals, improve discipline, control your habits and end procrastinating. How to achieve focus and find willpower and motivation as a way for success in your life

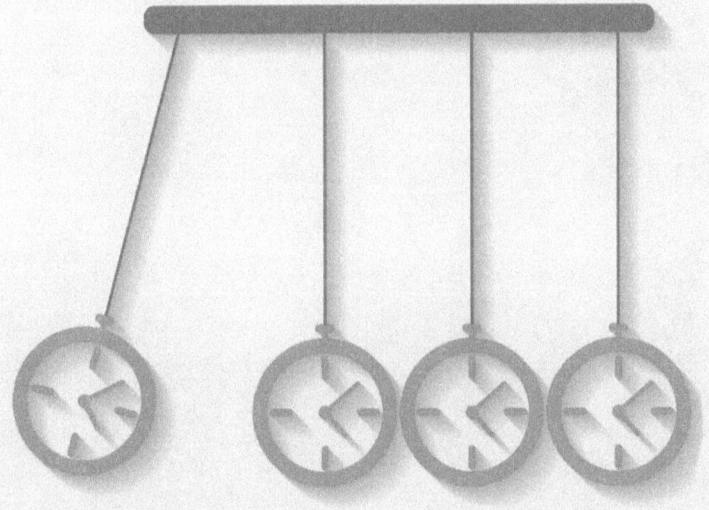

GEORGE M. POSI

BOOK 2: PROCRASTINATION

How To Stop Wasting Your Time And Be More Productive

Table of contents

HOW PROCRASTINATION SABOTAGES YOUR LIFE

E ven the most organized people do sometimes fritter away hours focused on trivial things like browsing on the internet aimlessly or binge-watching their favorite sitcom on Netflix when they know they should have devoted that very time to something more meaningful.

While on the surface, occasional procrastination is not that harmful, if you become a chronic procrastinator, then it negatively affects your productivity and, eventually, your prosperity and happiness.

Understanding the Basics of Procrastination

Procrastination simply refers to putting away a task for a later time. Therefore, if you are supposed to send an email to your boss, but you prioritize uploading your Facebook status over it, you are procrastinating on the former task.

That said, if you delve deeper into procrastination, you will realize that it mainly involves postponing a more critical task to do something less important, but seemingly more attractive.

Continuing with the example of emailing your boss, you find using Facebook, more entertaining than sending a work-related email, so you automatically lean towards the former task more even though you are aware of the importance of sending that email.

Occasional procrastination is not too harmful. Let's face it, all of us have resorted to it at some point in our lives and procrastinate on specific tasks even regularly. As long as that isn't affecting our lives negatively or does not keep us from achieving our targets set for the day, that's okay.

Procrastination becomes problematic only when we engage in it for too long and resort to it every time we have something incredibly important to do.

Let us look at the different ways through which procrastination harms you.

How Procrastination Sabotages Your Life and Wellbeing

- Lowers Your Productivity: One of the first and most substantial effects of procrastination is that it hampers your productivity. Naturally, when you keep putting off your work until the last minute, you keep piling up work, and when you finally start to work on a task, you have so much on your plate that you end up tossing the plate out the window instead of working on anything at all. This keeps you from achieving your goals and moving closer to the many goals you have in life.

- Affects Your Discipline: When you keep delaying your tasks, you soon inculcate the habit of procrastination. On the surface, this may not seem too disturbing to you, but deep down, it disrupts your self-discipline. When you keep giving in to your temptations, you soon let go of the inner resistance that helps you combat your distractions. With time, your ability to maintain self-control weakens, and before you realize it, you completely lose the discipline you once had to do what is right and essential.

- Weakens Your Self-Confidence: With time, procrastination starts getting the better of you and makes you falter at everything you do because you have lost the ability to work hard and believe in yourself. This depletes your self-confidence, and you stop trying your hand at things you really want to do.

- Increases Your Stress Levels: Stress is often rooted in the inability to perform as you do or not fulfilling your goals. Naturally, when you keep falling behind schedule, have tons of tasks to do, feel unconfident, and cannot muster the courage to battle your temptations, your stress levels increase, which adds to your problems.

- Affects the Quality of Your Life: If you are governed by your temptations and not your own will, you keep succumbing to your meaningless desires. Instead of doing what is right and important, you keep working on pointless tasks and never achieve the sense of contentment and fulfillment, you need to feel good about yourself. Also, procrastination gets in the way of your routine chores, personal goals, and your responsibilities towards your loved ones. All of this affects the quality of your life and keeps you from living a truly amazing life.

Simply put, procrastination does not help you live a worthwhile life. It gets in the way of everything you plan and aspire to do, which only adds to your misery. To gain confidence, nurture discipline, become healthy and develop grit so you can gather better control of your life and live it on your terms, procrastination is one unhealthy habit you need to break. Let us move on to the next chapter and find out the first step you need to take to move closer to this goal.

BUILD THE INTENTION TO BREAK PROCRASTINATION

E very journey to a goal begins with a commitment, a commitment to improving, to have better control of your nerves, and to work with dedication and perseverance towards the end goal to eventually actualize it.

Without a firm commitment and a clear intention to achieve a certain goal, you are quite likely not going to move dedicatedly towards it. This is why your journey to breaking procrastination needs to begin with an unwavering commitment as well.

Accept Your Problem

To build a clear intention to resolve your problem, you first need to admit that you have a problem to address in the first place. Unless you acknowledge your problem, you will not fully realize its effects on your life and will not work faithfully to fix it. Accepting your problem becomes more comfortable when you focus on how it is affecting (read: sabotaging) your life. To do that, do the following:

- Analyze your daily routine starting from the time you wake up until you fall asleep and list down all the tasks you actually engage in. Do write down the time you devote to every job.

- Now assess the importance of every task on the list and think about what it helped you achieve that day. For instance, if you spent 3 hours researching on your final year philosophy project in college, what outcome did you realize after that research? Were you able to carry out meaningful research, or were you not so pleased with your findings primarily because you did not devote 3 full hours to researching on the topic? Think about whether or not every task you do daily helps you achieve anything meaningful in the end. If your end goal for the day is to earn $100, are you able to do it considering the time you spend on your work-related tasks?

- Also, think about how much time you actually spend on the tasks stated on the list and how much of that time is invested in other activities. If you spent 2 hours drafting a 200-word email to a potential investor in your business, think about what you actually did in those 2 hours. Were you actually thinking about the content of the email and research on it to ensure you draft a well-structured and effective email, or did you spend 1.5 hours using social media on your phone and spent only 30 minutes doing the actual task?

- Moreover, think about the tasks you plan to do daily, but somehow end up not doing. Write down those tasks and compare their importance and the outcomes they would have helped you achieved with the functions already put on the list. If you had intended to write a blog post for your blog, email some PR firms, pitch a proposal to a potential client, do some household chores including laundry and preparing dinner and had to spend 2 hours with your family, but you ended up only writing a blog post and doing laundry, why do you think that happened? What went wrong, and where did it go wrong that made you mess up your entire plan and not achieve your set targets for the day?

Once you have detailed out all the answers to the questions and have analyzed your routine, go through the account a few times, and within minutes, you will realize how prone you are to procrastination and how harmful it is for you. When you compare the results you achieve every day with the desired outcomes, you will automatically realize how your habit to postpone essential tasks and engage in something less meaningful but more attractive while you are working on an important task is actually a destructive habit that is only destroying your life. This realization will help you accept your problem.

It is crucial to make a verbal and then a handwritten declaration of this acceptance to put things out in the open. Say and write down, "I have a bad habit of procrastinating on important tasks, and I am going to work to break this habit steadfastly." Your declaration can be different, but the gist of it should be the same.

Make a Strong Commitment Backed by Compelling Whys

Now that you have acknowledged your problem and committed yourself to fix it, you need to solidify your commitment and strengthen it by pegging it to a compelling why. You need to have a convincing reason or even several reasons why you need to overcome your bad habit of procrastination, so you work with dedication towards your goal.

The whys associated with every goal motivate you to work towards its fulfillment because they are the reasons why you are chasing that goal. If there is no reason why you wish to break procrastination, why would you ever do that? If losing weight isn't relevant to you, why would you ever hit the gym and focus on healthy eating? To overcome procrastination, you need to figure out exactly why you wish to do it.

Close your eyes, or even keep them open if you want and think about the most significant issue you are facing in your life right now. It could be anything that makes you feel discontent, brings you any sort of pain. Is it keeping you from living a completely comfortable and happy life? It could be your struggle with losing weight or the obstacles you are experiencing in setting up your business or how you are battling depression and the urge to give in to it or anything else that is seriously adding friction to your life and restraining you from living how you genuinely wish to live.

Write down your findings, and if you recall your work routine and how much time you spend on actually meaningful tasks and those that only make you waste time, you will realize that procrastination is indeed a primary reason why you are struggling to achieve your desired goals. Think about how your life would change for the better if you mustered up the courage to fight your temptations and beat procrastination to do actual work for real. Write down those reasons and use them to fuel your motivation to work towards your commitment to overcome procrastination.

Set a Clear Goal

Now that you have a clearer understanding of why you need to overcome your urge to procrastinate and are more determined than before to work towards this very goal, set a clear intention to actually beat this bad habit. You can have several goals on your list that you would like to fulfill to live a more meaningful, happy life, but it is quite challenging to work on a handful of goals at once.

Remember, you only have a certain amount of willpower to work on a specific task, and that willpower depletes with every move you make towards a particular goal. Therefore, if you work for 3 hours straight on creating your company's website, you are likely to feel exhausted after that and will not be able to work on another high priority goal for another couple of hours.

To ensure you don't run short of willpower to work on anything meaningful at all, go slow and steady. Do make a list of the goals you would like to work on to become active, enthusiastic, and productive, but pick one important one from the list that you would like to work on first.

Ensure to make that goal as clear and specific as possible, so you know exactly what you are trying to achieve. If your goal is to improve your income, think about the amount of money you would like to earn every month and compare it with the amount you are actually making. If you procrastinate on keeping your house clean, think about how clean you want your home to be, and create a specific goal based on it. Once you have better clarity on your goal, write it down on your journal.

You now have a compelling reason to overcome procrastination. Next, you need to make an action plan to work enthusiastically towards this goal and battle every temptation that comes your way. The next chapter shows you exactly how to do that.

CREATE AN ACTION PLAN TO WORK TOWARDS YOUR GOAL

'A goal without a plan is just a wish.'– Antoine de Saint Exupery

A the goal is actually quite incomplete without a plan of action. You can never achieve your goal unless it is accompanied by a plan. Not having an action plan is often the reason why people fail to achieve their goals and end up starting from point zero every now and then. If you don't want that to happen to you again, this time devises a detailed action plan before working on your goal just like that.

Figure Out Why You Procrastinate

To create a foolproof action plan, you need to figure out the areas that need your utmost attention and effort. For that, you need to identify the significant reasons why you procrastinate to know what keeps you from working on your goal and waste time on pointless activities.

- Do you put off important tasks because you find them challenging?
- Do you delay doing your work because you lack an essential skill that can help you perform effectively and efficiently?
- Do you procrastinate because you feel easily attracted to more attractive and relaxing tasks such as watching movies or napping?
- Do you delay working on high priority tasks because you are scared of faltering and failing?
- Do you procrastinate because you overestimate the time you have to work on a task and feel too confident in your ability to do it successfully on time?
- Do you delay your tasks because you somehow underestimate the time it will take you to complete them?

The answers to these questions will give you more precise insight into the reasons why you procrastinate so much. Often, a combination of all these reasons leads to procrastination, and often, there is a specific reason attached to the delay of a particular task.

For instance, you may delay working on your statistics assignment because you find the subject tough; but, you may end up not submitting your business proposal to a prospective client on time because you thought it would only take you an hour to draft it and you kept putting it off until the last minute only to realize in the end that you need at least 5 hours to work on it.

Think about the reason why you have been procrastinating on the respective goal that you have just set. List down those reasons and go through them a few times to better understand how they compelled you to put off your substantial tasks for a long time. You need to create your plan of action in a manner that all the duties and steps make you manage these reasons. Then you don't give in to them again.

Set Deadline and Incremental Goals

Next, you need to set a deadline to start working on your goal and another deadline on which its fulfillment is due. A starting date is essential so that you don't keep putting off the target until the last minute and can battle the reason for overestimating the time to work on a task. The ending date is crucial because it helps you know when the goal is due, so you don't waste another minute and get down to business right away.

Think about how much time you would need to work on your respective goal and consider the pace at which you work. Once you have analyzed these factors, set a starting and ending date, and write it down.

You now know when you must start working on it and have to complete it in due course. Your next task is to set incremental goals so you can systematically work towards its fulfillment instead of taking it as ONE, BIG Goal!

Often, people get intimidated by a goal because it is too big and feels overwhelming, even one that is spread over a month. 30 days are a lot also, you know! To keep this intimidating feeling on the sidelines only, set incremental goals for yourself to slowly adjust yourself to this new transition, and steadily move towards the end destination. For instance, if your goal is to complete your 50,000-word e-book that you plan to self-publish on Amazon Kindle, but you keep procrastinating on it, then your daily/ weekly incremental goals could be:

- Write 1000 to 3000 words in week 1
- Write 4000 to 7000 words in week 2
- Write 8000 to 11000 words in week 3
- Write a total of 15000 words in the next 3 days
- Write another 5000 words in the next 3 days to make 20,000

This way, you would slowly move towards your ultimate goal of writing a 50,000-word e-book and get done with your goal in 3 to 4 months.

Create a Working Strategy during Your Peak Energy Time

Next, you need to create an effective strategy that helps you work on your incremental milestones and achieve them. First, determine your peak energy time. This is the time of the day you are brimming with energy and have the zeal to work on even the toughest of tasks.

Observe yourself and how you work on different tasks for a few days, and you will start to notice a somewhat similar pattern in the way you work on various tasks at different times of the day. This will give you a clearer understanding of your peak energy time.

Your goal now needs to be to work on your incremental milestones during this time window. If, however, your peak energy time is just an hour or two-hour-long, you need to increase it. In that case, you need to start working in small installments of 2 hours, each separated by an hour-long break instead of trying to do everything at once. To increase your peak energy time, take things slow and easy, and don't fret on completing all your tasks in one go. With time, your willpower will improve, and you will slowly inculcate the ability to work for long.

You now have to draft a strategy on how to make the most of your peak energy time, so you get maximum output during that timeframe. Here is an effective plan that is quite likely to work in your favor:

- Think of the goal you plan to achieve during the first week. Having that in mind, identify the different things you have to work on to fulfill that milestone.
- Write down those tasks and then separate the high priority ones from the low priority tasks. The top priority tasks are all those that improve your productivity, and low priority ones are tasks that don't help you achieve your goals.
- Create a weekly to-do list that comprises of 4 to 5 high priority tasks that you have to do throughout the week to achieve your goal. Make sure the top priority tasks are assigned for your peak energy time.
- Break the weekly list into daily lists, and depending on your nature, pace, and the ability to handle different tasks, choose either of these two strategies. First, you do any one high priority and seemingly harsh task right when the day starts. This is also known as 'eat an ugly frog' strategy and is an excellent technique to kick start your day and boost your productivity. However, if that is too overwhelming for you, start with a seemingly more effortless task and gradually move towards a toughie at the end of the day or even the end of the week, so you have trained yourself to work consistently by then.

- Separate all your tasks with breaks in between so you get some time to rest and rejuvenate after working on an assignment for even an hour. Some people, especially those who have trouble concentrating on a task for even 30 minutes straight, work for 15 minutes then take a quick 5-minute break. You can even choose this strategy if it suits you. It is also known as the 'Pomodoro Technique' named after Italian chef Cirillo Pomodoro's tomato-shaped timer. Pomodoro is Italian for tomato. As the chef used his tomato-shaped timer to improve his time management skills and worked on 3 to 4 installments of 20 minutes each, the 'Pomodoro Technique' was created based on this. You also can work in this manner to make things easier for yourself.
- Identify all the probable distractions that lure you away from your essential chores and look for ways to manage them. For instance, if your hand unintentionally moves towards the TV remote every time you sit to work on your book, that there is your distraction that you need to overcome. If you are tempted to hit your snooze button and sleep for another hour every time you have to read articles for your thesis, that is your temptation that you have to work on. List down your distractions and look for effective ways to manage them. If you are tempted to sleep, maybe force yourself to get up and walk for 100 steps to charge up yourself, so you work on the high priority task. If the TV distracts you, take it off the wall and hide it in the attic so you have nothing distracting in your room and can focus better on working. Often, our distractions are associated with the environment we sit to work in. Bringing some changes in the surrounding is often the trick to manage distractions and increase our productivity.
- Next, you need to start working on the first task on your list and just do it without overthinking it. It is best to plan it beforehand right when you are creating your weekly/ daily to-do list, so you know how to execute it at that time. When it is time for you to work on your to-do list, pick the first task, and complete it right away. You don't have any time to think about it because that would trigger procrastination once again. Avoid that by just doing that task to save yourself from any trouble later on. If it helps, encourage yourself to work on it for 5 to 10 minutes only and keep going like that for a while. Referred to as the '5 Minute Hack', this trick mostly works well in helping you engage in a seemingly tough task and completing at least one part of it successfully.

Work on these guidelines consistently for a few days, and in a couple of weeks, you will get the hang of the routine and nurture a habit of it. You now have to keep working on your weekly to-do lists to achieve your incremental milestones, one after another, to move closer towards your destination.

Learn to Settle for Good Enough

Often, people who have the habit of chasing perfectionism and trying to do everything correctly, find it incredibly hard to achieve their set targets. If you are a perfectionist or use perfectionism as an excuse not to work on your plan of action, you are quite likely to fall in the same trap when you try to overcome your urge to procrastinate.

Now that you have learned how to commit yourself to this goal and know how to craft an effective action plan, you need to train yourself not to allow perfectionism to take over you.

To become a doer and achieve your targets, learn to settle for good enough results, and not exhaust yourself trying to achieve 100% results because nothing is really perfect. Perfectionism is a myth because nothing can ever be perfect. There will always be some room left for improvement, something that could have been better; some aspect that you could have paid more attention to and some area which, if you could have worked harder on, would have helped you achieve better results. The truth is this is because of a glitch in your mind. You need to fix that glitch to block your negative thoughts pertinent to overthinking and perfectionism.

Here is how you can learn to settle for good enough, overcome your tendency to chase perfectionism and slowly overcome procrastination for good:

- Whenever you start doing a task, think of the set target before tending to that chore.
- Go through the steps of the tasks and set a specific time limit to work on every level. If you have to create a business logo for a client and the steps involved include researching for inspiration for an hour, working on the logo for 2 hours, and making sure it complements the client's ideology and demands then make sure to work on every step for the designated timeframe only.
- Start working on the steps and make sure to spend only the designated time on every level, not even a minute more. If somehow you are unable to achieve a specific stage in the set time, move to the next step. If you cannot move forward without completing the previous step, take a break and tend to that chore after a few hours or at the same time the next day.
- Once you are done with a task, analyze your performance, and tell yourself how happy you are with the outcome even if you were able to achieve 50% to 60% of the set target. Smile and keep telling yourself repeatedly how pleased you are with yourself. If you do it intentionally a few times, you will eventually be happy

with your performance. That said, do identify your weaknesses and work on them to achieve even better results the next time.

If you consistently work on these steps and train yourself to achieve your set targets within the set timeframe and not spend extra time on a task, you will eventually learn to settle for good enough. Your next task is to further strengthen your focus, so you work with sheer dedication towards your objective.

REINFORCE YOUR FOCUS TO COMPLETE GOALS ON TIME

Your focus determines how far along you will move towards the pursuit of your goal like an anonymous quote states,

'When you focus on what you want, everything else falls away.'

If your focus is right and you are attentive towards precisely what you want, everything else on the sidelines stops distracting you. When you know you have to earn $5000 by the end of the month, you will not care whether you have to work for 6 hours a day or whether you have to work out in the cold. You know what you have to achieve, and you see nothing but your goal. This is the killer focus you need to actualize your goal, stay disciplined with temptations all around, and beat procrastination.

While the strategies taught in the previous chapters help you become focused, here are some more techniques designed primarily to sustain and increase your focus on your goal.

Visualize Achieving Your Goal

Visualization is an incredibly valuable activity that makes you consciously focus on your goal by training your subconscious to concentrate on the end goal. It requires you to imagine yourself achieving your goal. When you visualize yourself as a winner in your mind's eye, you train your mind to think positively. This creates many positive thoughts in that direction that draw positive experiences towards you, helping you achieve your goal.

Every morning when you wake up and each night before going to bed, think of your end goal and imagine that you have achieved it. Add as many details as you would like to add in this creative visualization and enjoy imagining that scenario for 10 to 15 minutes.

Also, slowly inculcate the habit to visualize yourself working on every task 10 minutes before doing it. So if you have to attend a seminar and present a speech on it, imagine you are at the venue and are delivering an impactful statement. This helps you map out the task in your head before actually doing it and trains your mind to work on it effectively, which increases your chances of success.

Visualization practiced daily helps you become an optimistic thinker and makes you hopeful of a bright tomorrow, which only improves your chances of success.

Become Process Oriented

As important as it is to be goal-oriented, it is equally important to focus on the process, the journey that takes you to the end goal. When pursuing a goal, we are likely to stumble and make a few mistakes. In that case, many of us often end up criticizing ourselves and quitting that goal altogether. This mostly happens because you fail to enjoy the journey that takes you forward towards your goal.

An excellent technique to ensure you aren't too harsh on yourself in difficult times is to become process-oriented. For that, you need to take an interest in every step of the process. Celebrate even your littlest of accomplishments to feel proud of yourself. Make sure to write down how you perform on every little to significant milestone and treat yourself to something nice every time you accomplish a set target even if it is something small as sending emails to potential clients. If you were able to do a task from your to-do list attentively and battle the distractions that try to entice you, you did a great job and deserve a nice treat to celebrate that. Also, every time you have a tough task on your list, set a reward beforehand. Indulge in that treat once you have accomplished that task to enjoy your accomplishment and the process that takes you to your goals.

Besides, track your performance to become better aware of your weaknesses and setbacks, so you improve on your shortcomings. Also, try different ways of doing the same task to find out the one technique that yields the best results. When you take a better interest in the process, you enjoy it more and happily work on even the difficult tasks to achieve your goal.

Steer Clear of Naysayers

One of the biggest distractions almost all of us experience is the naysayers around us. If there is even a single robust and negative influence in your life that keeps telling you how you cannot achieve your goal, that may be the reason why you fail to accomplish your goals.

When people keep telling you how your goal is way too difficult for you to accomplish; or how it is better to relax now and work later; or how you have been failing at achieving your earlier goals, so there is no point in setting more goals now, you are quite likely to fall in that trap. The moment you believe what the negative influences around you tell you, you trigger your habit of procrastination, and before you realize you are happily wasting away time doing pointless tasks.

If you want to stick to the routine you have created for yourself to slowly rid yourself of procrastination, you need to get rid of these naysayers from your environment to become more focused on your goal. Determine all these negative influences and how they impact you, and slowly distance yourself from them. Make a list of all the different people in your social circle, particularly those you spend the most time with. Think about the influence they have on you. Do you experience some sort of bitterness, negativity, frustration, and stress during or after you hang out with those people? Do you find yourself feeling demotivated and leaning towards your temptations and addictions after you have spent some time with some people? If yes, those people are the naysayers you need to reduce how much time you spend with them.

Being around naysayers only debilitates your self-confidence and sets off your tendency to lean towards distractions to manage your stress, boredom, and any other issue that you are going through in life. You really don't want that sort of negativity going around in your life because that only takes you away from what you aspire to achieve.

Now that you are well aware of how certain people impact you, slowly build the courage to distance yourself from them. Yes, you will have to be firmer with yourself and even with those people for some time, but with time and consistency, you will learn to manage the time spent with them and the way they influence you. You will have to stop taking the calls of certain people, block them on your social media, excuse yourself from particular social gatherings and make similar other changes to your routine and the way you interact with people to ensure you can block off their negative effect on your life. With some people, you will even have to be firm, but that is okay; you will see the fruits of doing this soon enough.

While you do that, surround yourself with positive people to feel inspired at all times. Just as negative influences distract you from your goal, positive impacts encourage you to work on your aspirations and nurture your motivation, enthusiasm, and a positive mindset. You need such influences in your life to arduously work towards the fulfillment of your goals and ardently work on your action plan to eventually overcome procrastination for good.

Also, look for any such person in your social circle who is working on a goal similar to yours, both the intent to overcome procrastination and the other purpose you have set to fuel your motivation to become disciplined. Ask that person to work alongside you so the two of you can serve as each other's accountability partners. An accountability friend is someone who keeps an eye on you, and your performance towards your goals keeps your triggers in check and motivates you to continually stick to your plan. This helps you manage your temptations successfully and do what is right. For instance, if you have a colleague who has been meaning to start his own marketing agency, but has been procrastinating on that task in one way or another, talk to him about your goal and work towards your respective goals together. This way, both of you can keep the other on his/ her toes and help each other in fulfilling your objectives.

Apart from doing the above, read positive books focused on self-development and listen to inspirational talks, podcasts and lectures on these topics to provide your mind with healthy mental food and encourage it to become more attentive towards your goal. You need to continually make sure that you think positively because if you direct your focus towards the right things, you gather inner courage to block all sorts of external negativity. When you are strong and optimistic for a better future from within, outside influences don't disturb you that much, and you can easily combat them. So ensure to read something positive every day, so you focus on your end goal.

Do Things You Enjoy

Also, to do all of the above, pay attention to your needs, and do things you actually enjoy. Often, procrastination is your way to vent out the in-built frustration because you haven't been able to do something you enjoy. If you have just been working hard for a long time and haven't done anything enjoyable for long, you are likely to lean towards meaningless activities. This can then trigger your habit of procrastinating and create more significant problems for you.

An excellent way to keep that from happening is to devote some time to your needs of enjoyment and entertainment occasionally. Make it a daily or weekly ritual to engage in some enjoyable activity such as painting, dancing, listening to music, or anything else that mitigates your stress and helps you breathe. When you consistently spend some quality me-time, you feel better and content with yourself and can quickly motivate yourself to work on your high priority tasks on time.

Remember, it takes time, courage, and perseverance to achieve your goal, so keep taking baby steps to climb up the ladder.

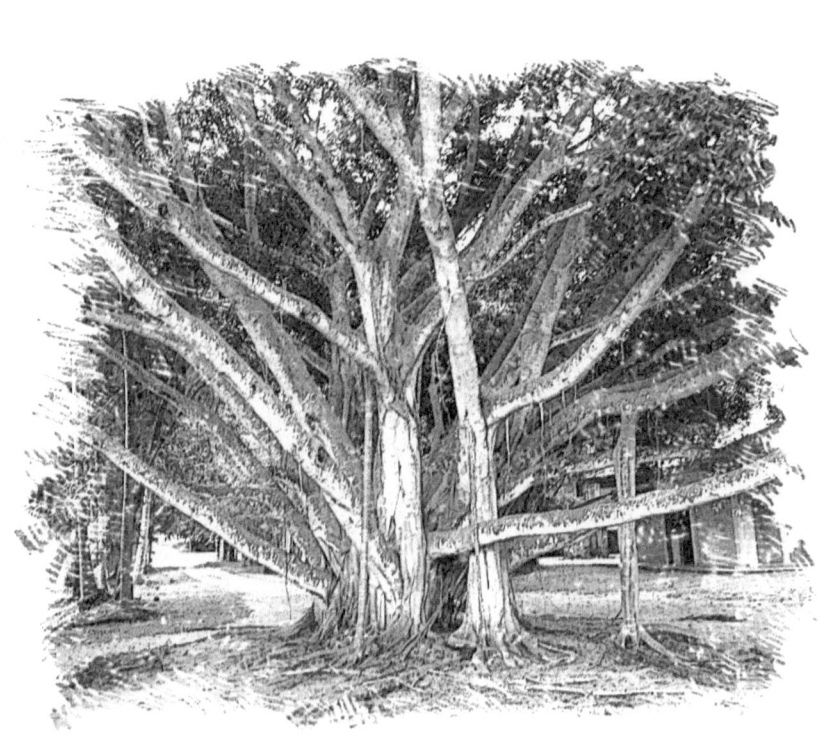

MINDFULNESS

THE BENEFITS OF MEDITATION, A BEGINNER'S GUIDE TO PEACE OF MIND IN YOUR EVERYDAY LIFE

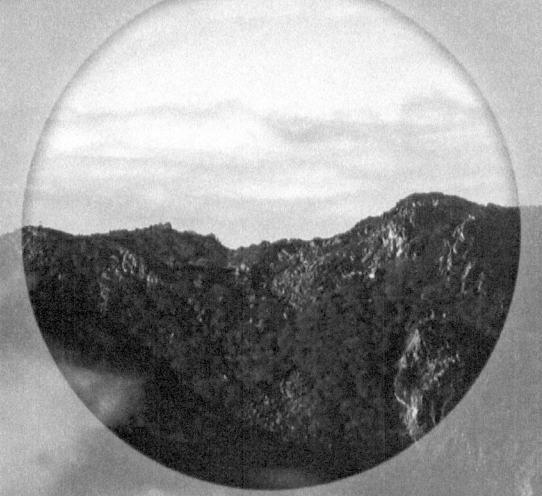

GEORGE M. POSI

BOOK 3: MINDFULNESS, THE BENEFITS OF MEDITATION

a Beginner's Guide to Peace of Mind in Your Everyday Life

Table of Contents

`

BUDDHIST PHILOSOPHY BASICS

Through its 2,500 years of existence, Buddhism has had time to develop many different nuances. Buddhism teaches us not to just accept things blindly but, rather, encourages us to challenge and test every claim stated in its teachings. It is best to apply this attitude to every word in this book as well. Blind faith is not a good practice. Learn to just have an open mind, and you will see for yourself. The best way to investigate your personal discovery is through meditation.

Pain and worry are of great concern in your life. If you wonder where the pain comes from, then maybe you have failed to observe the world as it really is. You adopted some mental constructions as "me," "the table," "the house," and you presumed that those were solid, real entities. You believed that they would last forever. They never do. All of reality is in a state of constant change. Observe how your life is in the ever-flowing movement. All you need is to put some effort and time into it. You should use this insight as an experience of impermanence and unsatisfactoriness.

You may worry a lot. Worrying itself is the problem. Anxiety is a process that you build in your mind. It starts as the grasping/rejecting reaction. As soon as an object of anxiety pops into your mind, you often try to mentally hold onto it or push it away. But the Buddhist way is to see things as they really are. If you deprive objects of their seeming permanence, then you can see that this worry will also pass.

If you, through practicing meditation, demystify this illusion, then your whole universe changes. It is a long process, so do not expect to be able to do this right away. For the mind map that you spend your whole life building, it will take some time to change. Meditation is a process by which you will be able to do this. With mindfulness meditation, you will learn how to see what you are doing, when you are doing it, and how you are doing it. You are now in a position where you can decide to do it or not, whichever seems appropriate to any particular situation. Instead of being compulsive, you now have a choice.

For these significant insights, you may need to put considerable effort into the practice of mindfulness meditation. It is not easy; it is not fast. But eventually, it pays off. Pushing this practice all the way will enable you to achieve your well-deserved mental health, a true love toward all beings, and the end of suffering. That is no small goal.

Although this can take a lifetime to accomplish, some benefits start right away and increase over time. The more hours you spend on mindfulness meditation, you gather more ability to be calm and observe your impulses and intentions as you become more involved in your regular meditation practice. You will be able to have better insight into your thoughts and emotions, the moment they form in your mind. On the same token, you can stop during the process any time you feel you've had enough. You will still feel the difference.

Achieving peace and happiness

Peace and happiness are really what all of us are looking for. On the surface, it seems that you want food, wealth, sex, entertainment, and respect. In the end, it all comes down to peace and happiness.

Then, you can ask, what is happiness? Is it to have everything you want and to be in control of everything? Think again. Are the people that have control and power happy? Well, not more than others, really. It is not possible to have everything you want. Instead, you can learn to control your mind, to stop being contaminated with desire and aversion. You can learn to recognize desire. You can also learn not to be controlled by it. In no way does this mean that you should lie down and accept everything that happens to you. It just means that you assume a new point of view on everyday life events. By all means, you will change things that you can, but you will also learn to accept those that you cannot.

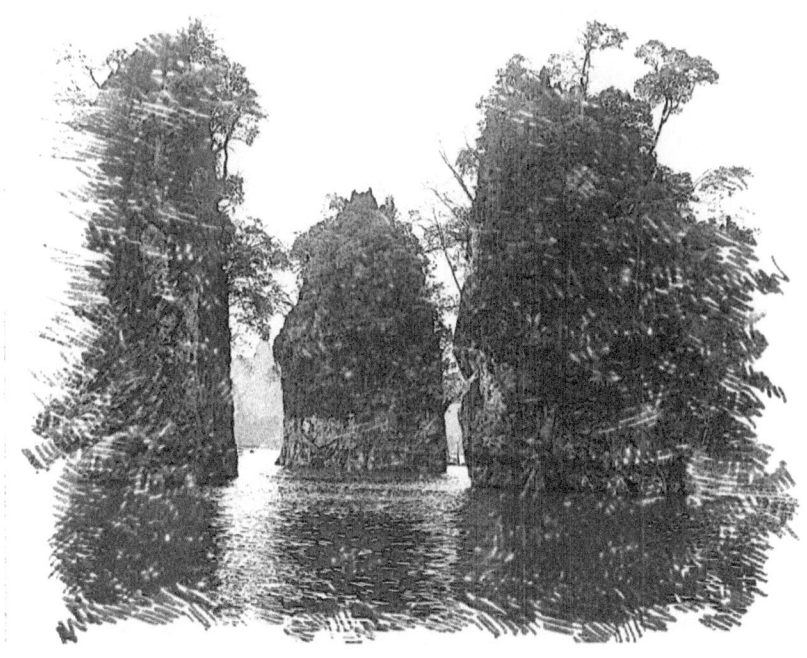

Look carefully inside yourself, truthfully and objectively, and learn to see those moments. Learn to see them without judgment, and you will be able to make radical changes in your everyday life. Then, you will see yourself as you are right now. You must let go of all illusions, judgment, or resistance to change. You will, of course, stay active in society as the social being you are. You fulfill your duties and obligations to your family and friends, and to all fellow human beings and, most importantly, your responsibility to yourself. This is your path to achieving true happiness.

As your understanding grows, the more compassionate you can be. You will be ready to forgive and forget and to learn to love by understanding. This is only possible if you understand yourself.

This is not an issue of faith. This is an issue of confidence and experience. It is made through everyday practice and endurance on the path to discover things as they really are.

An attitude toward material necessities

Some material necessities make your life possible. There is no need to refrain from them and become ascetic, but you really need to keep them on a level that will not become excessive.

You should eat food that is food, not just "bait." Eat food for the proper nourishment of life.

You should wear clothes that fulfill the real meaning and purpose of clothing: good health, protection against annoyances and discomfort, convenience and simplicity, and expression of culture.

The shelter should be adequate, modest, and not excessive. Nowadays, many people live in homes that exceed their needs, are very expensive, cause worries, and lead to frustrations. Unfortunately, housing becomes a source of much selfishness.

One of the most critical life conditions is medicine, which I think needs no further explanation.

Then there is an indulgence. You can stay a part of the community, and still, have your needs fulfilled with non-material and non-lustful things. Of course, you can be a great person who caves into those from time to time. You just never should hurt others to do so.

The Four Noble Truths and The Eightfold Path

If you want to have a deeper understanding of why mindfulness meditation is so successful and has been a significant part of the lives of many people for thousands of years, it is better to explain some of the basics of Buddhist philosophy that this whole concept is based on.

This philosophical construct is based on what Buddhists call "The Four Noble Truths" and "The Eightfold Path."

The First Noble Truth, with its three aspects, is: "There is suffering, dukkha. Dukkha should be understood. Dukkha has been understood."

It is essential to understand that Buddhism is not telling you that everything in life is suffering. Just that there is suffering in life.

"Dukkha" can be translated as "incapable of satisfying," always changing, incapable of truly fulfilling us, or making us happy.

One more important detail is that it says: "There is suffering," and not "I suffer." This non-self approach is crucial in understanding the essence of Buddhist philosophy.

Our goal is to see or accept things as they really are.

The term "suffering" refers to things that you usually do not want to know or feel. When you are in situations that you don't like—that is suffering. On the other hand, you may want to hold onto something beautiful because you don't want to be separated from it. But all of us and all things—the whole of life is impermanent. You will be parting of all of those things eventually. It is essential to know and accept this.

The Second Noble Truth states that there is an origin of suffering and that the root of suffering is attachment to the three kinds of desire: the desire for sensual pleasure, the desire to become, and the desire to get rid of something.

If you, let's say, enjoy eating chocolate, then you want more, and you often cannot stop. Sometimes, you get caught in striving to become happy, seeking to become wealthy, or hoping to maybe become something other than what you are right now.

On the other hand, maybe you want to get rid of your anger, jealousy, fear, or anxiety.

There is nothing wrong with those wishes. The problem arises when you start to identify with desires in any way, and they begin to control your life. But desire has power over you and deludes us only if you grasp it, believe in it, and react to it.

When you contemplate desires and accept them, you are actually no longer attached to them. You now just allow them to exist as they are. At that moment, you learn that the origin of suffering and desire can be laid aside and let go of.

But how do you let go of things?

It is essential to acknowledge that "letting go" is not "getting rid of'. " If you are holding onto something and you say, "Let go of it! " that doesn't mean "throw it out. " Thinking that you must throw it away would just be the desire to get rid of it.

It is crucial to know when you have let go of desire. Only when you no longer try to get rid of it will you know you are ready to leave the desire behind you. Then, you recognize that it's just the way it is. When you are peaceful and calm, then you will know that there is no attachment to anything. You are not trying to get something or trying to get rid of something. Knowing things as they are in the crucial step for letting them go.

The Third Noble Truth is: "There is the cessation of suffering, of dukkha. " In this sentence is the essence of Buddhist philosophy. The aim is to develop a reflective mind in the pursuit of letting go of delusions.

The mind should be in a mental state that can accept the way out of suffering. It is no longer a mind that has prejudices and thinks it knows it all. This is now the mind that is open to these Four Noble Truths. Your mind can now reflect on things that you can acknowledge through conscious thought.

When you meditate, before you can let things go, you have to skilfully allow the subconscious to rise into consciousness. All your fears, anguish, despair, and anger are allowed to become conscious.

This is the most important path that you must walk by yourself. No one can do it for you. You need to be determined and not give up.

The Fourth Noble Truth says: "There is the Eightfold Path—the way out of suffering."

You can divide the elements of the Eightfold Path in three groups:

The first group consists of Wisdom (pañña), Right Understanding (Samma Ditthi), and Right Aspiration (Samma Sankappa).

The second group describes Morality (Sila), Right Speech (Samma Vaca), Right Action (Samma Kammanta), and Right Livelihood (Samma Ajiva).

The final group includes Concentration (Samadhi), Right Effort (Samma Vayama), Right Mindfulness (Samma Sati), and Right Concentration (Samma Samadhi).

The list above does not mean that elements of the Eightfold Path will arise in this order. The fact is that they all happen at the same time. Presenting them in this order simply teaches us to reflect upon the importance of taking responsibility for what you say and do in your life.

The first element of the Eightfold Path is the Right Understanding. It comes to us through insights into the first three Noble Truths.

If you have these insights, then you understand impermanence. "All that is subject to arising is subject to ceasing." It is a simple but powerful truth.

As you meditate, you experience calmness, and the mind slows down. When you look at things with a calm mind, you are looking at it as it is. Then, there is nothing to gain or get rid of. It is precisely what you see; you are not criticizing it, comparing it, or trying to possess or own it. It is precisely what it is.

The second element of the Eightfold Path is the "Right Thought"—more precisely, you aspire to think in the right way. It is essential to acknowledge that aspiration is not the same as desire.

Taking responsibility for your speech and being careful about what you do with your body represents the moral aspect of the Eightfold Path. The Right Speech, the Right Action, and the Right Livelihood are parts of the moral dimension of the Path. This means that when you are mindful and aware, you speak in a way that is appropriate to the time and place. You also act or work according to time and place.

Sticking to those morals, you will begin to realize that you need to be cautious about what you do and say. If not, you will just end up hurting yourself. Saying hurtful things will always have an instant result, even if you can't see it right away.

If you do things without any personal desire for gain, just because it is the right thing to do, then you are on the right path to gain your peace of mind.

For everyday life, the Right Livelihood is essential when you come to know your intentions for what you do. Then, you can try to avoid intentionally harming other beings or earning a living in a damaging, unkind way. In your contemporary understanding of this Path, you also try to avoid becoming addicted to alcohol or drugs. You will be cautious and avoid actions that might endanger the ecological balance of the planet.

The Right Action, the Right Speech, and the Right Livelihood are natural extensions of Right Understanding. You will begin to feel that you want to live in a way that is beneficial to the planet or, at least, that does not do harm to it.

The Right Effort, the Right Mindfulness, and the Right Concentration are the qualities of your spirit and your heart. These three are integrated together and work toward achieving the goal of supporting each other. No one is dominating the other, nor exploiting or rejecting anything.

Deploying the Right Effort, you do the best you can, but you also realize that it's not up to you to do everything and make everything right.

If you have the Right Effort, the Right Mindfulness, and the Right Concentration, then you are fearless, because there is nothing to be frightened of. The strength of your morals encourages you to do good and to refrain from doing evil. This is a perfect path because everything is helping and is mutually supporting: the body, the sensitivity of feeling, and your intelligence. They are all in perfect harmony.

What is Nibbana?

Nibbana is probably the most popular but most misunderstood term in Eastern philosophy. In Theravada Buddhist tradition, "Nibbana" means "coolness." The most significant benefit of mindfulness meditation is that you can achieve Nibbana right now, without having to die.

It is important that you correctly understand the word "Nibbana." It means "cool" or "the absence of heat." It has nothing to do with dying. Imagine that everything is going right for you: you have good health, economic security, great family, best friends, and pleasant surroundings. In this interpretation of Nibbana, this life of yours is "cool." It may not be perfect, Nibbana, because to be accurate, it must include a cool mind, but it is cool just the same.

Do not worry too much about reaching Nibbana. It will come to you eventually. The path to it will have great value as well.

MINDFULNESS MEDITATION

What is meditation?

H uman beings can make their minds stable and focus. This enables us to make the full use of it to understand, to think, and to create. To fully develop those capabilities, you have to practice letting your mind to grow. You can learn to be mindful, to be concentrated, and to understand, but the mind will not fully develop without proper mental exercise.

The technique to develop these qualities is called "meditation." When you meditate, you explore yourself and try to grasp how the mind works. You use a technique to develop your mind, the same way you use physical exercise to build your muscles.

Every day, thoughts just come into your mind. There is rarely the intention of thinking. It is just a waste of your mental energy. You get exhausted after only half an hour of being engaged in wandering thoughts. Meditation will help you to put those thoughts away. Sometimes, you cannot even sleep because your mental energy is used on those unwanted thoughts. Frustration and agitation also waste your mental energy. Eventually, that will also affect your physical health.

It is essential to learn how your mind works in everyday situations, not only when you feel angry, agitated, unhappy, but also when you feel happy. You meditate explicitly to learn those things about yourself. When you know about your disappointments, resistance, resentments, and frustrations, you can accept them and then get to know them more intimately.

This will enable you to understand how your mind works.

How does meditation work?

The English word "meditation" does not enclose all Buddhist ideas represented in the Pali word "Bhavana," which means "to develop the mental ability."

Meditation is not just about to be willing to sit quietly, closing your eyes, thinking only of what is right in your life, and ignoring all that is bad, cultivating an optimistic view. It is not the case that meditation has little to do with your everyday life. It is not only for monks and old people who have retired and have time for it. Meditation could, in some religions, also mean reflection on past events, your right, and poor deeds, etc.

For successful meditation, you must first accept how you perceive the world around you. In Buddhist teachings, there are six senses. You learn about the outside world through the eyes, ears, nose, tongue, body, and mind. The first five are physical senses, but the mind is a mental sense. Things you perceive through your six senses are meditation objects. Things that come into your mind are also meditation objects.

Concentration

Having just one mind, you can only focus on just one of those objects. This is the reason you need to learn meditation techniques.

The way to be focused on just one object is to "close the doors" for others. This is what you can call "concentrating." You focus on only one object or one point. Sometimes, this is called "One-pointedness."

During the day, you want to do so many things. But thinking about all of them simultaneously will get you nowhere. You need to develop an active mind to be able to enjoy your surroundings and, ultimately, your life. You need to have a sharp mind and decide on just one at the time. This will enable you to enjoy your current activity. This is the foundation of concentration.

Breathing

Your breath is almost the only sure thing in your life. It is with you as long as you live. You can rely on it. It will always be your retreat from all your hectic surroundings.

Begin by focusing your mind on your nostrils. Start breathing in and out regularly. As you breathe in, say, "breathing in..." As you breathe out, say, "breathing out..." Your mind will go somewhere, often repeatedly. Just take note of the place it went and repeat its name. Then, return your focus to your breath. It is also the same for the feelings that could arise, external distractions, etc. You just notice them, repeat in your mind what the distraction is, and gently remind yourself to return your focus to the breath.

Pain

During meditation, the idea is to sit still. In most cases, you are not accustomed to sitting in a meditation posture for a long time. Pain might arise. This pain is not here to punish you nor to make you uncomfortable. It is just a natural consequence of you not being accustomed to this sitting position. Also, this pain will teach you how to deal with pain in general, in your everyday life.

Here's what you should do when you feel pain during meditation: when you feel pain, let's say in your knee, you switch all your mental energy to your knee. Register it in your mind as "pain, pain, pain." Then gently go back to breathing. The pain may increase or decrease. If the pain increases, go back there again and repeat "pain, pain, pain." Try to stay with what comes in your mind because of that pain. It might be agitation, impatience, frustration... Say all of them three times, then go back to your breath. The pain can then increase or decrease. Eventually, if the pain becomes too unpleasant, just mindfully change your position and go back to being focused on your breath.

DIFFERENT FORMS OF MEDITATION PRACTICE

Mindfulness with breathing meditation

One great experience I had was my visit to Wat Suan Mokkh, where I participated in a 10-day meditation retreat. I have described my experience attending the retreat itself in my blog post, Ten Days Of Unforgettable Experience: Meditation Retreat, and now, I would like to reflect more on the teachings that I received there. It had a profound impact on my life, so maybe it can help you as well.

The foundation of the teaching is complete dedication to "Anapanasati-Bhavana" (mindfulness with breathing) meditation.

The correct and complete practice of this kind of meditation is to take some truth or reality of nature and then observe, investigate, and scrutinize it in mind with every inhalation and every exhalation.

In this type of meditation, you will contemplate the secrets of "kaya" (body), the secrets of "Vedana" (feeling), the secrets of "Citta" (mind), and the secrets of "Dhamma" (the teaching of Buddha). These four objects' secrets should be accepted into your mind and then studied.

You start with a breath. There are different types of breathing: long breaths, short breaths, calm breaths, violent breaths, fast breaths, and slow breaths are different types. You need to analyze, to examine the nature, characteristics, and functions of each kind of breathing that arises. Also, you learn how different breaths have different effects on your body.

While you are getting ready to start your meditation, first, you must choose a place that is suitable and appropriate for the practice. The site does not need to be perfect because you cannot find such an area.

This place just needs to be quiet and peaceful, where the conditions are right and where there is the least possible disturbance. But if that is not available to you, then you can focus on the breath and be aware of other external conditions so that you can accept them. Also, whenever possible, you should choose a time of the day when there are no distractions or disturbances. But this is rarely the case, so you should just use the best time available.

There is also the consideration of a teacher. A good teacher can help, but you should not forget that no one can directly help someone else.

Next, you need to assume the appropriate sitting posture. It is essential to sit in a way that is both stable and secure, so when the mind becomes semiconscious, you will not fall over. It is also important to sit upright, with the vertebrae and spine in proper alignment, without any bends or curves. The vertebrae should sit snugly, one on top of the other, so that they fit together correctly.

At first, keep your eyes open, gazing toward the tip of your nose so that your eyes do not get involved with other distractions. If you close your eyes, you might get sleepy, so be careful about this option. Later, as you gain more experience, you will be able to meditate even with your eyes closed.

You will now come to nothingness, contemplating your breath, and developing "Sati" (mindfulness or reflective awareness) by being mindful of each in-breath (inhale) and each out-breath (exhale).

Let it be natural. Do not interfere with it in any way. Then, contemplate each breath with mindfulness. How are you breathing? What is exhale like? Note your observations so you can compare them with your later experiences.

Next, find a place where you can easily observe your breath. In the beginning, take a few deep, steady breaths, to find and keep this spot. It can be the tip of your nose or your lips. Once you find it, observe that point as the breath passes in and out. The breath becomes subtler and gentler as soon as you start to note it and follow it.

Finally, when you stop chasing after your breath, it calms down even more. You can verify this through your own experience.

It also helps to count. You can count each inhalation as it starts, one number for each breath. If the mind wanders, start counting again. If you can count to ten without the mind wandering, go back to the beginning anyway.

These tricks will help you get started. When you adopt them, you will always have them at your service in your meditation and in your everyday life.

Now, when you settle into observing your breath, you can expand this a bit more.

Become aware of the three primary segments of each breath: the beginning, middle, and end. You will feel them during the inhalation in your nose, the middle of the chest, and the abdomen, and then the reverse during exhalation. This way, you will have a better understanding of your breath, and when you master this, you can move your focus to other challenges, like your feelings and your thoughts.

This is something I will leave for the next book.

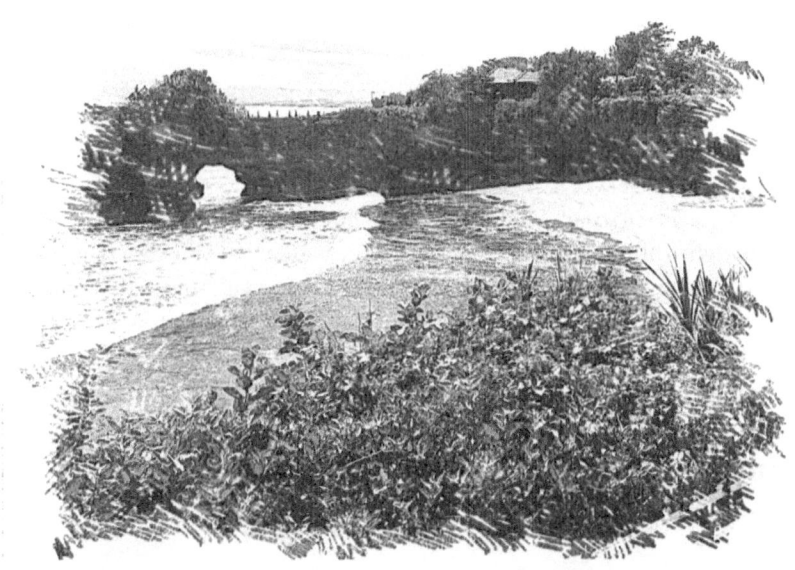

Metta meditation

I will now explain how to perform Metta meditation. Let me first say something about the purpose and meaning of this type of meditation in Buddhism.

"Metta" can be translated from Pali (the language of Buddha) as "loving-kindness" or "friendly love." Many Buddhists regard this type of meditation as the default kind. Metta meditation is constructed of four components: Metta, "Karuna" (compassion), "Mudita" (sympathetic joy), and "Upekkha" (balanced mind).

In my next book, I will go more in-depth about the Buddhist view of origins, as well as reasons why Metta meditation works. I will also explain the terms mentioned above. For now, let's just learn some proven techniques on how to do successful Metta meditation.

For beginners, it is best to concentrate only on the Metta part of contemplation and meditation. The rest will follow if you persist with the practice.

Metta represents the desire to see peace and success in your life, as well as to be free from harm. This then extends to members of your family and friends, and later, it becomes universal.

Prejudice and fear are the manifestations of opponents of Metta. Anger and ill-will have destructive forces within and without.

Metta meditation cannot be performed in the absence of mindfulness. You must have sustained awareness while practicing meditation that's focused on breath before you are capable of doing Metta meditation.

For Metta meditation to be successful, you must have been engaged in putting forth the right effort. You must really mean the words that you are saying to yourself while meditating. Developing Metta is, therefore, crucial in overcoming frustration within oneself. This gradual reduction of frustration is the first benefit that one earns from Metta meditation.

How to practice Metta meditation

Metta meditation is often performed toward the end of your awareness of breath meditation. Leave the last ten to fifteen minutes to reflect on your Metta thoughts.

You should now contemplate some unfavorable conditions that you do not want in your life and some favorable conditions, feelings, or things. Contemplate on desirable and undesirable events happening to you. For example, I have a headache, and sometimes, I cannot sleep. I have met these difficulties, and I have become mindful of these difficulties. With a feeling of Metta for myself, my first wish is that I may "get rid of the headache."

On a more positive side, I wish that to become more successful in my blogging and book-writing. These are my two most important things nowadays. I will incorporate them into my Metta practice.

First step

In the beginning, choose yourself as the meditation object. Repeat to yourself in your thoughts, "May I be free from (state first negative condition). May I be free from (other negative condition). May I be able to (state first positive condition). May I be able to (other negative condition)." Repeat these two to five times.

Second step

Now you can direct your thoughts to a person you care about—such as your parents, children, spouse, or siblings—then visualize them and repeat: "May they be free from (say your choice of one negative condition). May they be free from (say your choice of a second negative condition). May they be able to (say your choice of a positive condition). May they be able to (say your choice of a second positive condition)." You can wish them to be free from illness, and to have good health, or some more specific condition that you know is appropriate for them.

In this way, you will develop mindfulness of your feelings of wellbeing, your desire to be free from harm, and suffering, and this then leads to the development of Metta for yourself and the people closest to you.

Third step

Now, you choose a neutral person. They may be someone from work or someone you have come across anywhere you've gone, someone you neither like nor dislike.

This person is entirely neutral. Direct your Metta thoughts to that person in the same way as you did before.

In your first Metta meditations, do not use the people you have been in conflict with or had arguments with. Do not start with people of the gender you're attracted to, as this can provoke lust. Also, do not use those who have died, for this can stir up sorrow.

You can also have the next part of Metta meditation directed to an unspecified person (your whole country, world, any other living being, etc.). You can try this in your next meditations.

Vipassana meditation

The purpose of meditation is to clear your mind and get rid of greed, hatred, and jealousy. Meditation helps you to bring your mind to a state of concentration, insight, and tranquillity, and as a consequence, you can achieve awareness.

If you seek personal transformation, you should try to meditate. It will help to change your character by setting your mind to become calm and still.

Meditation helps you to reduce restlessness, tension, fear, and worry.

It will not alter your reality; it will just help you to see the world as it is. You will still be exposed to the pains of life, but you will now understand them and thus be better able to handle whatever misery comes your way.

Meditation is a slow and subtle process but offers real liberation if done correctly. This is something that you must achieve by yourself. Retreats, books, and teachers might help, but this is ultimately your path.

"Vipassana Bhavana" is a term for insight meditation in the Pali language. "Bhavana" means to cultivate the mind. "Vipassana" is derived from the word "Passana," which means seeing or perceiving. "Vi-" is a prefix that can be approximately translated as "in a special way." So, vipassana Bhavana implies the cultivation of the mind toward the aim of seeing in a single direction that leads to insight and complete understanding. It is also known to be translated or explained as meditation for the sake of insight into impermanence, unsatisfactoriness, and not-self.

You would like to practice vipassana meditation to help you to be able to face reality or to experience life just as it is. Then, you cope with what you discovered.

When practicing vipassana meditation, you will not forget or put aside your problems. You will see and accept reality as it is. After that, you can change it.

Vipassana is the oldest of Buddhist meditation practices. It comes from the Satipatthana Sutta, which is thought to have been told by the Buddha himself. Vipassana is a direct development of mindfulness or awareness.

When you practice vipassana meditation, your attention is gently directed to a holistic examination of aspects of your existence. You are trained to observe more and more of the flow of your life experience.

Vipassana is very, very hard to do, even if it seems very gentle. It trains your mind to focus on attentive listening, mindful seeing, and careful testing. You will be able to "smell actually, to touch fully" and notice the changes that are taking place during these experiences.

Very important is that you learn to listen to your own thoughts without being caught up in them. That way, you will see the truth: objects are impermanent and unsatisfactory.

Vipassana is a process of self-discovery, an active investigation in which you observe your own experiences while participating in them.

If you pursue your meditation practice with an open mind, you will succeed.

By practicing vipassana meditation, you will be able to condition yourself to see reality truly as it is. You will gain mindfulness.

Throughout your whole life, you try to make yourself feel better and happier. You desperately try to put away your fears and gain security. At the same time, real-world experience is not affected by your wishes. When practicing vipassana meditation, you will learn to ignore your urge to live a luxurious and shallow carefree life, and you will be ready to accept reality. Then, you will be able to choose your battles wisely. Another interesting fact is that, often, real peace comes as soon as you stop chasing it.

If I can now conclude what vipassana meditation represents for, I would say that it is a set of practices that open us, step by step, to a better understanding of reality as it truly is, how things actually feel. For me, the most significant advance in my knowledge of vipassana meditation is that it teaches you to stop thinking about life; instead, you just live it fully. Vipassana will guide you to live in this moment because the past has already happened, and the future is yet to come, as Buddha said. So, make most of this moment, and don't spoil it with endless regrets or by dreaming about a future that might never happen the way you hope it will.

There is not some unique technique to it. You are practicing vipassana as you are focusing on breathing, just you now letting all of emotions, feelings, and thoughts to arise. You acknowledge them, accept, and then let them go. It is much easier to write this down here than to practice, but with all the insights you learn from this book, it will get more comfortable every time. You just need to sit and genuinely commit to doing vipassana meditation. I will be going more in-depth in some subtleties of vipassana practiced in one of my later books.

Other forms of meditation

Meditation is not only limited to the Buddhist tradition. Although techniques in different religions and cultures are enormously varied, and there are many forms of meditation or contemplative practice, they all can help many believers or non-believers to achieve their peace of mind. I will describe, in brief, a few.

Within the Judeo-Christian tradition, there are two leading practices: prayer and contemplation. Prayer can be described as an address to God.

Contemplation is a process of conscious thought about a specific topic; religious ideal or religious script. Those are exercises in concentrating. That will mean that the mind is brought to one aware area of operation. The positive effects are that you can find a deep calm, a physiological slowing of the metabolism, and a sense of peace and well-being.

Hindu tradition nurtures yogic meditation as purely concentrative. It focuses the mind on a single object, not allowing it to wander. In advanced practice, yogis proceed to expand it by assuming more complex objects of meditation.

In addition to concentration, Buddhist meditation aims at the development of awareness, using focus only as a tool toward that end. Zen Buddhist meditation uses two separate approaches.

The first is the direct dive into awareness by pure force of will. The aim is to just sit down and throw everything out of your mind — everything except the pure consciousness of sitting. This is very hard to achieve.

The second Zen approach is to trick the mind out of conscious thought and into pure awareness by having a student to solve an unsolvable riddle, thus placing him in a terrible training situation. Even if Zen is helpful to a lot of people, it is very tough.

On the other side of "toughness" is tantric Buddhism. So, there are many ways to achieve peace of mind. You should never believe blindly, but try it yourself and figure out what feels right for you.

MINDFULNESS MEDITATION IN EVERYDAY LIFE

Most of scientists in any article agrees that mindfulness meditation has a profound effect on your body and mind. Some of the well-described benefits are made through improvements to your well-being, increasing your chances of leading a satisfying life. Being mindful not only enables you to enjoy good things fully in life as they occur and helps you to be truthfully engaged in activities, but it also increases your ability to deal with undesirable events. By focusing on the here and now, you are accepting that the past is gone, and the future is yet to come and is unknown to us. Remember, this does not mean you shouldn't plan for the future, or that you shouldn't learn from the past. It only means that you should work on the things that you can influence and that you should accept those that you cannot.

Mindfulness, especially in combination with yoga or another physical activity, improves physical health. Mindfulness can help relieve stress, sometimes lower blood pressure, and reduce chronic pain. It can also improve sleep.

Mindfulness improves mental health, reducing your risk of depression, substance abuse, eating disorders, and anxiety.

How to Practice Everyday Mindfulness

It is hard, but still easier to practice mindfulness meditation in your quiet room than to adopt that mindset in your everyday life. In sitting meditation, you can use the anchor for your attention by developing the awareness of one particular part of the experience at the moment, such as breath awareness.

That anchor helps you to see when the mind has drifted away to some other area. By contrast, in everyday life, you do not have such reminders; you have no peace of mind to remind you to be mindful. Instead, you are often distracted by daily events. You need an anchor point.

How do you choose a reference point to serve as your anchor? It is best to choose an activity that you regularly perform, something you do every day, and several times a day. The simpler, the better. There are many things to do, say, 3-4 times a day. For example, you can choose the moment of passing through a doorway or picking something up. When you start working with a reference point, you'll probably miss it a lot of times before you remember it. You may remember your tasks only in the evening when you lie in bed.

It's not a problem if you do not think about it at any point in the day, and then it comes to mind in the evening. That moment is the same as when you realize in sitting meditation that the mind has lost its breath. Then you know: "I am here now, and I forgot to do what I intended." This moment is not proof that you are unable to practice, but just the opposite! Because at that moment, your exercise just started. So, look at what is happening right in front of you, without disappointment or self-judgment.

When you go through the door, just observe that at this moment, you are going through the door. Awareness can be extended for a few seconds after that, but do not ask too much of yourself.

One of the best areas for exercising intent is speech. Paying attention to what you are saying can be a massive challenge. Often, you speak automatically, without even considering what you are about to declare. It is a good practice to stop before you talk — take a moment's break. You should remember to stop! Then you will be able to recall that you will say something, that all speech has intentions, and if you are careful during this break, you have the opportunity to, firstly, look at what you will say, and secondly, what motive is behind it.

Then you will know clearly what your motives are and when they will not produce the desired result. This should not be a source of self-criticism and self-control, but rather an opportunity to learn from the moment. Thus, when you realize that some motivations will lead to pain and suffering, for you or for others, you will have the choice to leave it behind.

The present moment is the only place where you can decide what will be your answer to what life puts before you. The past is irreversibly behind you; there is no more, except for memories in your mind and this very moment. The future doesn't exist either, except as thoughts in the present moment. So, all this exists only now, created through a mixture of causes and conditions, most of which you cannot control either. The one and only choice that is under your control is your reaction here and now.

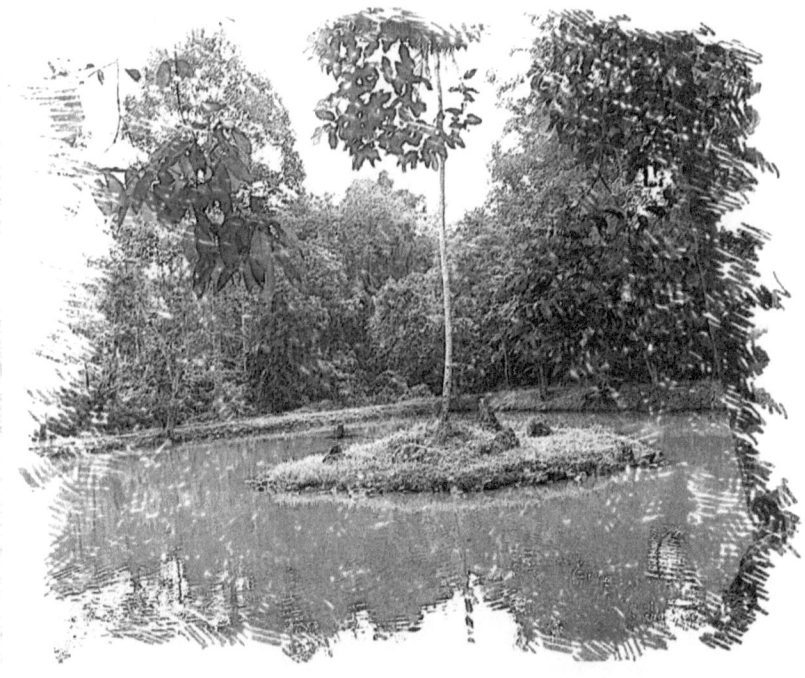

When you notice that your mind begins to preoccupy you with thoughts of the future or the past, gently restore it to the present moment by looking closely at the sky or the people around you.

Practice enhancing your awareness, for example, by waiting until the phone rings three times before you answer. Be aware of the jobs you are doing: making your bed, washing dishes, getting dressed, etc.

Even though the reward is valuable, it is a big challenge as well. Thus, it is necessary to arm yourself with patience. Countless times, you will realize that you have forgotten to do that. Be compassionate toward yourself. Be persistent in your practice, and you will eventually succeed, because what is the alternative? Even more absence and distraction? Your determination will slowly begin to break the barriers of unconscious habits and patterns of thinking that keep you separate from reality and far from the truth of the present moment, and far from yourself.

* * *

Just be mindful and do not give up.

PROCRASTINATION *Cure*

HOW TO USE MINDFULNESS MEDITATION TO STOP PROCRASTINATING

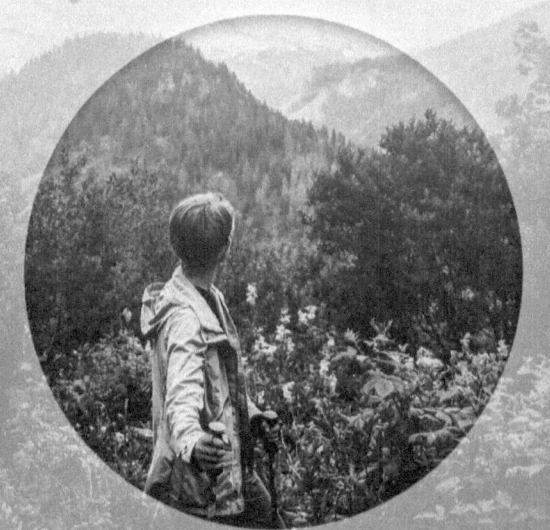

GEORGE M. POSI

BOOK 4: PROCRASTINATION CURE

How to Use Mindfulness Meditation to Stop Procrastinating

Table of Contents

WHAT IS PROCRASTINATION?

Procrastination is putting away a task for a later time. Therefore, if you choose to check your Instagram before you start doing a business report, you are procrastinating.

When you dig deeper into procrastination, you will understand it means delaying a more critical task to do something less important, but apparently more attractive.

The term "procrastination" means a complex disturbance in the process of controlling the action and is associated with low self-regulation capacities. Arguably, the group most affected by procrastination is students. It is said in the Study done by (Höcker et al. 2013) that 75 percent of them report being obstructed by procrastination.

We all procrastinate from time to time, and as such, procrastination is not too harmful on that scale. It is important not to let it affect our lives negatively. It must not influence our mind and keep us from achieving our daily tasks.

Procrastination becomes a problem when it persists for too long and kicks in every time we have some vital tasks to complete (or even just to start).

Procrastinating is "killing" productivity and is a significant concentration inhibitor. Engaging with the activity that has been put off often leads to stress and poor performance.

Procrastination is a fascinating topic, especially regarding the online world. Are you pushing something important to a later time just by reading this?

If you really looking to improve yourself and are deliberately seeking a book like this, then please do read on.

Why Do We Procrastinate?

Our brains receive a reward for avoidance when we procrastinate (The Psychology of Procrastination, Jackson Brammer, M.D., David Puder, M.D.) It delivers instant relief from the discomfort connected with the task. Sometimes, we may feel uneasiness just moments before an assignment is due, but we rarely think about the past or the future when procrastinating.

Procrastination, therefore, creates a cycle that wears down our self-confidence. It plays with our subconscious mind and puts a burden of guilt and regret on us.

Effects of Procrastination

Procrastination harms you in many different ways. Thoughts and emotions tend to just pop up out of nowhere. It is in their nature. They appear, and then they disappear. It is just like that.

Similarly, negative thoughts and emotions will pop up when you need to even start a challenging or uncomfortable task.

Negative thoughts and emotions will appear when you are trying to finish your assignment, meditation, workout, or, in fact, anything meaningful. Then you feel stressed out, overwhelmed, and anxious. For sure, you don't feel motivated. Your mind is suggesting that you do the task tomorrow. Tomorrow, you will feel like it, and tomorrow, you will be motivated.

Your mind will rationalize and come up with a perfectly good reason for avoiding anything that is even slightly unpleasant, and it creates endless excuses as to why you shouldn't do something now. Surely, those reasons are irrational, but they sound superficially reasonable.

Do you experience some of these thoughts? Of course, you have. These thoughts and the emotions that go along with them are what lead us to procrastinate.

It is always the mind — our thoughts and emotions — that gets in the way. When you want to meditate, or even get up early, your mind tells you to start tomorrow. It is much more fun to watch YouTube the whole time and go from one suggested video to another until you are so tired that nothing else matters.

Fortunately, there is a solution. Thoughts and emotions don't need to determine your behavior...

Feelings and thoughts often determine the way we act; we make changes to our posture, voice, facial expression, and practice. This is called an "action tendency." But it is just the tendency.

We do have the inclination to do something, but that doesn't mean we have to do it. We can feel afraid but act courageously; we can feel angry but act calmly; discouraged, but keep going, nonetheless. Despite feeling negative emotions, and have negative thoughts, you still can do what you need to do. You can do this even if you don't feel like it.

Scientific Research

Timothy A. Pychyl, the author of Solving the Procrastination Puzzle, defines procrastination as a self-regulation failure. (Dr. Pychyl is an Associate Professor in the Department of Psychology, the Director of the Centre for Initiatives in Education.)

We tend to go into so-called "task avoidance" mode whenever we are faced with tasks that prompt any kind of negative emotional response, especially feelings of frustration or boredom. This is particularly true if we have low self-regulation. We tend to say to ourselves that we will do this later or that we'll do it after some other, more pleasant task. We cannot just acknowledge and move past our feelings of wanting to do something else. We are compelled to immediately act on them.

Procrastination is not just a problem when it comes to getting things done. We tend to lie to ourselves about how we really feel and are more likely to have compulsive behaviors or develop addictions.

Procrastination is not something we are born with — it is a learned behavior — so we can act to ignore the urge to put off a task when we feel unpleasant emotions. Pychyl states that "effective self-regulation relies on emotion regulation, and this emotion regulation, in turn, relies on mindfulness."

Being mindful of this moment right now will bring some instant benefits, but only if we practice it persistently can we master our thoughts and emotions. This will help us become more and more sensitive to the subtle emotions that come and go throughout our day.

Michael Inzlicht is a Professor of Psychology at the University of Toronto, where he is also cross-appointed as a Professor in the Rotman School of Management. He has studied prejudice, academic performance, and religion, but his most recent research is focused on the topic of self-control. He writes, "Mindfulness as a practice cultivates the ability to maintain focus on the present moment. This present-moment awareness provides sensitivity to sensory cues—like that negative emotional pang we might feel when facing an aversive task."

Mindfulness has an excellent advantage if we implement it. Then, we begin to notice when we are starting to feel uncomfortable, bored, frustrated, or even scared by a task. Then we can kindly recognize and accept the feeling and make a conscious effort to stay in control. It will not always be successful, but with awareness comes the choice to do things differently. So, it is worth the effort, because success will not simply arrive overnight.

Compassion and acceptance are also crucial parts of mindfulness. Inzlicht and Rimma Teper concluded that people who were better at controlling their behavior were probably able to do so because they were "more accepting of their errors and associated conflict."

For long-time procrastinators like myself, it can be challenging to get into a mindfulness meditation practice at first. Over time, I have become aware of my resistance. I learn to accept it, and I notice what feelings arise when I begin to meditate.

To delay action for a while is not problematic. The conscious decision to prioritize what you need to do is a self-regulation act. But if this action is not performed, but some less necessary task is, then this behavior becomes problematic.

According to Rückert, procrastinators are more likely to experience stress, a loss of time-management, irregularity in their actions, and negative feelings about their procrastination behaviors. About 75% of college students report that procrastination behaviors deter their studies (Höcker et al. 2013). Steel (2005) found that 95% of students describe themselves as procrastinators with motivation and a desire to reduce conduct.

Baumann & Kuhl (2013) found that internalization can enhance intrinsic motivation through self-knowledge, which can be supported by meditation. Meditation practitioners show more activation at the anterior cingulum, which leads to the conclusion that meditation practitioners have more attention regulation and are less easily disturbed (Purdy, 2013).

People that practice meditation improves their ability to arrange their ideas and thoughts. Through meditation, they can see clearly what they want to do or what they need.

The study "Meditation and Procrastination" (M. Thyea, K. Mosena, U. Wegerb and D. Tauschelbsuggests, 2016) shows that quantitative results indicate that the participating students who are experienced in meditation show a very low score on procrastination. In conclusion, that mediation is associated with lessened procrastination, with possible mechanisms of increased acuteness of thoughts, the focus of attention, and self-regulation.

It is no surprise, then, that 75% of the participants related the effects of their meditation practice on their learning behavior with their ability to manage their time. By practicing meditation regularly, they increased their general reliability, regularity, and structure.

The results deliver evidence for the theoretical connection between procrastination and meditation. The meditating students participating in this research study showed extremely low levels of procrastination.

In the study, as mentioned above, the participants described that their self-regulation mainly influences their attention regulation, the regulation of emotions (like anxiety), and their self-perception. Procrastination is about the intention to fulfill a task, and instead of fulfilling the intended task, they perform another, mostly unimportant task. If the alternative job is perceived as more attractive, and the intended one as aversive, then procrastination is more likely to occur.

The students who meditated seem to be able to focus their attention better on an intended task and don't feel disturbed by alternative jobs. They felt more self-confident and experienced less anxiety, which is another explanation for procrastination among students (Höcker et al., 2013). The participating students explained that using meditation strengthened their emotional regulation. Disturbing emotional states are perceived as less disruptive, and by controlling their focus of attention, meditating students can stick to their planned tasks and do not get caught up with alternative tasks.

MINDFULNESS IS A STATE OF MIND

Mindfulness is, no doubt, your most potent weapon in the battle against procrastination. The Oxford Dictionaries defines mindfulness as "a mental state achieved by focusing one's awareness on the present moment, while calmly acknowledging and accepting one's feelings, thoughts, and bodily sensations, used as a therapeutic technique."

Keeping a non-judgmental, moment-by-moment awareness of events in the present moment is mindfulness. Awareness of bodily sensations, thoughts, feelings, and the environment is the essence of mindfulness. The non-judgmental part means that we pay attention to our thoughts and feelings and just accept them without judging them. We do not put the label of "good or bad" or "pleasant or unpleasant." Instead, we only observe.

Mindfulness allows us to acknowledge our thoughts and emotions from a distance, but not identifying with them. It will enable us to feel negative emotions without having a reaction to them.

Mindfulness and Emotions

I often wonder how life would be if I could better manage my emotions. Is the path to a happier life just getting rid of your emotional side, or is the solution something much deeper? Buddhist philosophy offers one possible explanation, as well as suggestions, for how to live a balanced life, with emotions that are not going to make you unhappy.

In the framework of Buddhist meditation or meditation insights, when it comes to emotions, we choose the middle path. We neither suppress them nor encourage them and manifest them. We do not ask ourselves to deny them, nor do we act according to their dictation. We simply allow them to go their own way through our body, mind, and heart.

There are three essential components of each emotion:

· Thoughts: a story, a trigger for emotion.

· Physical sensations: how the emotions manifest in the body. Every emotion has its own tangible counterpart.

· Emotional state: can be subtle or completely obvious. Something similar is when we put color-tinted goggles, which then can make our experience frightening. Fear has one color; joy has another.

When we are aware, we can notice each of these components. The thought or story often inhabits us, and we lose focus. It is, therefore, often useful to try to distance yourself from thoughts related to your emotions.

Regarding procrastination, mindfulness allows us to act even if we have negative emotions. We get the opportunity to do the right thing, regardless of how we are feeling at that moment.

Mindfulness will make you happier, healthier, more self-compassionate, more self-disciplined, better at tuning out distractions, and much more.

All of the things mentioned are countless times proven to influence procrastination by lowering it. This, in the end, will make you a better student, teacher, or entrepreneur.

Research has shown that mindfulness is an effective strategy for dealing with procrastination.

My own experience supports this in full, though everyone's experience is different. I think that mindfulness is the most essential skill we can ever learn in our lives. Regarding procrastination, I felt great benefits from mindfulness. I've become aware of my thoughts and emotions. Mindfulness enables me to deliberately choose if I will react or not. This way, I can stay with my feelings and thoughts, let them be, while I'm completing the task ahead of me.

As my friend Stephanie pointed out to me recently, it is possible to use meditation to actually procrastinate. Of course, meditation is an excellent tool, but like any tool must be used in good faith and responsibly. So, we will put this issue aside for now.

For sure, mindfulness improves my self-control, makes me aware of myself, and diminishes feelings of guilt for procrastinating occasionally. For me, it is clear that mindfulness is one of the most precious remedies for curing procrastination.

The benefit of having emotions is that they provide us with information. Emotions are also adaptive. We now understand that emotions have motivational properties. Although a task ahead might evoke fear of failure, other emotions set up task aversions, such as boredom or frustration. These emotions motivate us too. They can motivate avoidance or procrastination. We must be aware of emotions so that this awareness can invoke self-regulation, rather than avoiding what needs to be done.

Mindfulness is more than awareness, however. Mindfulness also includes the critical feature of non-judgmental acceptance of our emotions (or thoughts).

When we can cultivate mindful awareness and acceptance, we then can understand our motivation to procrastinate and to exercise the control that is essential for staying on the course until the initial emotions pass.

By including mindfulness practices into our daily lives, we can nurture a compassionate awareness that is the solution to procrastination.

Maria Konnikova (Russian-American best-selling writer and psychologist) describes procrastination as "an impulse that requires self-regulation." She stated that "those of us who are genetically hardwired for impulsivity and spontaneity are also more likely to procrastinate."

Suffering

According to Buddhist philosophy, our goal is to see or accept things as they really are.

The term "suffering" refers to things that you usually do not want to know or feel. When you are in situations that you don't like, that is suffering. On the other hand, you may want to hold onto something beautiful because you don't want to be separated from it. But all of us and all things, the whole of life is impermanent. You will be parting of all of those things eventually. It is essential to know and accept this.

If you can accept that suffering is inevitable, putting it off starts to make much less sense.

The modern world places overwhelming challenges on us, enabling, or even encouraging, procrastination. Look on the Internet. It has become the most effective enabler of procrastination. It goes along with the behavior of a distracted mind. It predicts what we are likely to do or to see, just to avoid things we do not like to do right now. The Internet is designed to occupy your mind with short content that ends before your mind gets bored, so you can quickly move on to something else.

How we waste time may have changed, but procrastination existed long before the Internet. The fundamental impulse to do so is just as accurate as it ever was because it relates to the basic urge to avoid suffering. It is the nature of thought and feeling. Putting stuff off originates from this same desire to move away from suffering. But if you can accept that suffering is inevitable, then putting it off starts to make much less sense.

You need to give these ideas the benefit of the doubt and just try to practice some mindfulness meditation exercises. If you can recognize the moment you are about to begin doing something for the sole purpose of avoiding doing some important task, you'll often find the need to do so really subsides. This is one of the things that a meditation practice can help with. Giving you enough perspective on your thoughts is a step in the right direction. It can be relatively easy not to act on the impulse to procrastinate. All you need to do is nothing, not to give in to the urge to start some meaningless activity.

It is always easy to find a reason why we're procrastinating. We don't want to go to work, or to clean our house, or to study for pointless exams, we just don't want to complete our tasks every day. Even when we think we know why we're avoiding tasks, the real reason might be a little more complicated.

It is known that procrastination is often a mechanism for coping with the anxiety that is associated with starting or completing any task or making decisions. In that case, it is even more essential to adopt the practice of mindfulness, as a way to be aware of our wishes and duties, and to find the strength to complete them.

There is also a matter of duty. Unlike negative connotations that this term brings in Western civilization, the term "duty" in Buddhism is tied to our inner feeling of obligation to ourselves and the duty to fulfill our purpose. This subtle difference means a lot. If we feel that completing our commitment is a part of our purpose, we will be less likely to procrastinate on accomplishing them. When you can adopt this stand, it will make things much more apparent to you.

Stress

We cannot concentrate when we are stressed. Stress is a part of life, and thus, we have to find a way to manage it effectively. We will find that the cause of stress is typically associated with work, school, family, relationships, and financial issues. While stress undoubtedly plays a role in our lives, we do not have to allow it to take control of our lives. Even if it is hard to believe right now, we can choose how to deal with stress and stressful situations. We can effectively manage stress, also though we cannot eliminate it completely.

It is well-known that stress is a part of life. We recognize three types of stress: physical, nutritional, and emotional. We will focus here on emotional stress.

Emotional stress is one that you can effectively manage through mindfulness meditation. It will enable you to live happily and healthily by getting a handle on the things that stress you most.

Awareness of Your Emotions

One of the best ways to stay aware when there is a strong emotion is to stop and notice how it affects the body, to connect with the physical sensations associated with emotion, turning our attention away from the emotions. Otherwise, emotions, especially strong emotions, are very seductive and a powerful magnet for our attention. Sometimes it seems like they are commanding us: "Pay attention to me!"

We are used to sensing our emotions in the way that they occupy us completely. If we learn to pay attention to emotion in a different way, we can treat it with due respect, but not to be trapped or blinded by emotions.

For example, if we are angry with someone, we usually focus on the person, and in our head, we rewind the film countless times to remember and think about what this person did to us.

In our mind, instead of paying attention to a person or a situation, we should carefully look at this experience of anger. Instead of focusing on the outside, we should focus inward.

The practice of Emotional Awareness

In your everyday meditation, as described in my book Mindfulness: Yoga And Meditation, Simple Beginners Guide To Stress Relief And Happiness, when it comes to paying attention to emotions through our practice, we should say that we are not looking for certain emotions during this practice. Instead, the basic instruction is to keep your focus on your breath.

We give priority to the physical sensations caused by our feelings. But if some emotion comes up and starts to require your attention, then leave your breath aside and focus on the bodily sensations provoked by that emotion instead.

When these sensations are no longer dominant, gently return to your breath. If the emotion is so strong that it makes it impossible for you to be with your breath or body, direct your attention to that emotion itself. See if you can identify and name it. Let it go. After some time, the feelings will fade, so you can return to your breath.

Experiencing Emotions

Emotions want to be experienced, but if we stay with the object of emotions or their story, it gives them all new strength. At the same time, this prevents us from feeling complete. But if we turn to the emotions itself, to the physical sensations they cause, and to the effect that comes to mind, then the emotion has the chance to live its life more naturally. And it will, usually, sooner or later, reach its end. As is the case with all other phenomena. Its energy is not infinite.

Everything emerges, stays for a while, and then disappears forever. Emotions are no exception.

Conscious emotions need you to let them manifest themselves in their natural and healthy way. But that does not mean that we become their "soldier," to do what they tell us.

Tools for Dealing with Emotions

We can use four tools to help us deal with emotions: recognition, awareness, exploration, and non-identification.

Recognition

Sometimes, it is quite clear to us what we are experiencing, and it is easy to name it: rage, happiness, loneliness, or fear. When we are aware and clearly recognize and call an emotion, we are actually unbinding the knot in which it tied us. Sometimes, it takes time to discover which emotion it is; we are not always clear on which one, but we do know that we're experiencing something!

Sometimes, we have the feeling that this is a mixture of emotions, where none of them are dominant. In that case, it is enough if we only register emotion, confusion, or one of the more broad categories: chaos.

Permission

In the context of meditation of consciousness, every emotion is acceptable. You can give yourself unconditional permission to have any emotion. There is no need to censor or criticize your feelings. Practicing meditation is an entirely safe place to let yourself feel what you are experiencing. Since you've decided to sit still during meditation, you've given up the idea of doing what your emotions are instructing you to do instead. It's effortless, so just stick with it.

Sometimes, we want to get rid of unpleasant feelings as soon as possible. But if you try several times, you will discover that emotion and uncomfortable feelings will completely fade and disappear. This experience is one of the most inspirational in the entire practice of meditation. It also gives us a powerful emotion that we, not our moods and emotional states, can manage and control our lives.

Exploration

Through awareness, we learn to explore the experience of emotion at the present moment. How do you know that you are experiencing a specific feeling now? What does it say to you?

Do you feel anger, joy, depression, or surprise? In searching for such signals, it is best to turn to your body, as emotions usually have physical manifestations. There are many physical feelings that emotions can cause. Anger can result in stiffness and heat.

Fear can cause a stomachache, and joy can produce a faint flicker throughout the body.

These physical feelings associated with emotion are not stories that take place in our minds but are rather physical experiences of the present moment. The best way to get away from the story, which usually refers to the past or the future, is to focus on physical sensations and thus bring us back to the present moment.

Non-identification

Usually, we tend to identify ourselves with our emotions. We think they display and represent who we really are: I am a person who often runs away; I am a depressed person; I am a happy person; I am a fearful person. All these conditions and moods, we consider essential parts of our being. When emotions take hold, there is always some kind of identification with it, a feeling of an "I," "me," or "mine" identification with a story related to that emotion.

All the tools, as mentioned above, help us by bringing our mind and body into one point, which is the present moment, by stabilizing our attention on the "now."

Working with Positive Emotions

The most disturbing emotions are painful emotions. When meditating, we hope to get feelings of peace, tranquillity, happiness, balance, bliss, and joy. It's good to work with those emotions. It is important here to pay attention to the tendency to identify with them. When happiness arises, our reaction may be an attempt to keep it. Maybe we think, "This should always be the case. Now I finally understand how to practice this practice. I will never be unhappy again..."

It's easy to become fascinated by pleasant emotions, staying blind to the fact that we are increasingly immersed in emotion. This type of reaction can be the cause of later disappointments, when feeling fades, as is the case with everything. In time, we will discover that those emotions are even more fulfilling when we do not identify with them. They become even more satisfying when we are not attached and afraid to lose them eventually. We must be aware that all emotions, bad and good, also will pass. This is a truly liberating feeling.

A MINDFUL APPROACH TO PROCRASTINATION

Procrastination is just one of the many ways we use to avoid discomfort, and it is ubiquitous. We can become very skilled at avoiding pain. Avoiding unpleasant feelings is a very human thing to do, but, unfortunately, not all discomfort can be avoided.

Organizing a life that minimizes our contact with things we don't like is our aim. Sometimes, though, disappointments and losses cannot be avoided. It is essential to learn how to manage those, because if we are not trained at handling frustrations, then we easily get overwhelmed when difficulties arise. We don't have a strategy for dealing with the discomfort, and we do not believe that we can cope with various challenges that arise inevitably.

Mindfulness meditation helps build your capacity for tolerating unpleasantness without getting overwhelmed. If you are always avoiding discomfort, your ability to hold painful feelings gets diminished, but when you practice accepting suffering, then you can manage a higher degree of discomfort without your mental health being threatened.

For all the years I have been practicing meditation, I was able to develop the skill to accept events in life that I personally do not like, and that causes stress to me. That way, the impact that stress has over me is much more manageable and is not felt or interpreted as a threat to my well-being.

For me personally, learning to let go has been one of the most tangible benefits of my meditation practice. I have developed the skill of sitting quietly and watching the way my feelings come and go away. If I just breathe and observe, things move on. It is very dangerous to get caught up in negative thoughts and endlessly repeat them in your head.

But, it is possible to just let them go. Watch your breath. Maybe other thoughts will arise; perhaps they won't.

Just observe. These thoughts are not what define you or your life. They are just a moment in time that you can let pass. I am not saying it is easy; I am saying that practicing mindfulness meditation is worth the effort to try.

How does this help with procrastination? Procrastination is often triggered by negative thoughts. These thoughts lead to anxiousness and are of no practical use when completing a task. Our first action is usually to try to avoid them by avoiding our work.

With mindfulness directed toward these moments, you are aware of the thoughts coming up and how anxiousness arises. You will also become mindful of the feeling of your feet on the floor of your breath going in and out. This puts those negative thoughts on the same plane as others, and they lose their significance. They are just thoughts passing through.

Do not get involved with negative thoughts; just leave them alone. Tolerate the discomfort while remembering it is only natural to have those thoughts. But now, you are not controlled by them. You can instead turn your attention to the task ahead and start to work.

It takes some practice, and you will really learn your whole life, but in time you are no longer getting caught in negative thoughts. You now can move on.

Procrastination always boils down to that decisive moment when we're facing a task: we can either do the thing, even though we don't feel like doing it, or we can run away and procrastinate.

Clearly, reducing long-term procrastination means getting better at resolving this situation. We become able to act despite experiencing negative thoughts and emotions.

The mindful way of thinking enables us to watch our thoughts and emotions from a healthy distance, being indifferent to them as much as possible. You will develop this ability more if you practice it regularly. Mindfulness allows you to see your negative emotions without overreacting to them.

Mindfulness is crucial in overcoming procrastination, and it is one of the most important skills we can ever learn. Mindfulness as a way of conducting your life is a great tool to overcome procrastination. It will help you to successfully manage your thoughts and emotions in everyday life.

Mindfulness is much more than a passive meditation. We learn how to observe and accept our emotions as a cognitive skill. You can use it to create new forms of behavior that will help you accomplish your long-term goals.

It is important for the mind to fully attend to what is taking place, to what you are doing, and to space through which you are moving. Every so often, we veer from the issue at hand; our mind takes flight, we stop being in touch with our body, and we slowly become absorbed in obsessive thoughts about stuff that has already taken place or continuously worry about the future. That creates anxiety. Yet, regardless of how far away we drift, mindfulness is there to take us back to where we are and what we are feeling and doing.

Bottom line: mindfulness itself is the practice of focusing all your attention on the present moment purposefully and accepting it resolutely without judgment. It's a perfect place to begin if you are looking for true peace and happiness.

MINDFULNESS MEDITATION

Mindfulness meditation is a powerful ancient technique that has been used for years, mainly to reduce stress, anxiety, and depression and to achieve inner peace. It has also been used to relieve pain and treat certain illnesses. But what exactly is mindfulness meditation?

Mindfulness will help you identify cognitive distortions, thus being an efficient way to avoid procrastination. Trough gentle observation of mindfulness, we become aware of the problem. This is the prerequisite for change in our thought patterns. Mindfulness makes us aware of our overall behavior.

Mindfulness meditation re-trains your mind to remain in the "now" or present moment, entirely calm as it should be. Many times, we become anxious and stressed because of a disturbing past that we keep thinking about or worrying about a future that you have no control over. With mindfulness meditation, you learn to live in the moment, as that is the only thing that you can change — you have no control over your past or future.

While its exact origin is still somewhat vague, the practices and instructions of mindfulness meditation have been found in the ancient texts of several major religions such as Judaism, Buddhism, and Hinduism. Even so, Buddhism plays a pivotal role in helping us understand the concept of mindfulness meditation; the practice is integral to the "Buddhist path."

In Buddhism, cultivating non-judgmental awareness of yourself, your feelings, and your mind is considered very important.

When practicing vipassana meditation (Buddhist form of mindfulness meditation), you will not forget or put aside your problems. You will see and accept reality as it is.

Buddhist Meditation

The English word "meditation" does not enclose all Buddhist ideas represented in the Pali word "Bhavana," which means "to develop mental ability."

Meditation is not just about to be willing to sit quietly, closing your eyes, thinking only of what is right in your life, and ignoring all that is bad, cultivating an optimistic view. It is not the case that meditation has little to do with your everyday life. It is not only for monks and old people who have retired and have time for it. Meditation could, in some religions, also mean reflection on past events, your good, and bad deeds, etc.

For successful meditation, you must first accept how you perceive the world around you. In Buddhist teachings, there are six senses. You learn about the outside world through the eyes, ears, nose, tongue, body, and mind.

The first five are physical senses, but the mind is a mental sense. Things you perceive through your six senses are meditation objects. Things that come into your mind are also meditation objects.

Buddhist Concentration

Having just one mind, you can only focus on just one object. This is the reason you need to learn meditation techniques.

The way to be focused on just one object is to "close the doors" for others. This is "concentrating." You focus on only one object or one point. Sometimes, this is called "One-pointedness."

During the day, you want to do so many things. But thinking about all of them simultaneously will get you nowhere. You need to develop a strong mind to be able to enjoy your surroundings and, ultimately, your life. You need to have a sharp mind and decide on just one at the time. This will enable you to enjoy your current activity. This is the foundation of concentration.

The basis of Buddhist philosophy and understanding how the world works is described in Four Noble Truths and The Eightfold Path.

The First Noble Truth, with its three aspects, is this: "There is suffering, dukkha."

It is essential to understand that Buddhism is not telling you that everything in life is suffering. Just that there is suffering in life.

The Second Noble Truth states that there is an origin of suffering and that the root of suffering is attachment to the three kinds of desire: the desire for sensual pleasure, the desire to become, and the desire to get rid of something.

The Third Noble Truth: "There is the cessation of suffering, of dukkha." This sentence is the essence of Buddhist philosophy. The aim is to develop a reflective mind in the pursuit of letting go of delusions.

The Fourth Noble Truth says, "There is the Eightfold Path — the way out of suffering."

You can divide the elements of the Eightfold Path into three groups:

•　The first group consists of Wisdom (pañña), Right Understanding (Samma Ditthi), and Right Aspiration (Samma Sankappa).

•　The second group describes Morality (Sila), Right Speech (Samma Vaca), Right Action (Samma Kammanta), and Right Livelihood (Samma Ajiva).

•　The final group includes Concentration (Samadhi), Right Effort (Samma Vayama), Right Mindfulness (Samma Sati), and Right Concentration (Samma Samadhi).

We will now focus on Concentration (Samādhi). The correct concentration is the last member of the noble eightfold road. This means that there is a wrong concentration.

In Buddhist teachings, concentration is a neutral function of the mind that exists in every state of consciousness. When the mind focuses on one single object, it provides a subjective experience of exceptional inner peace and, in the end, silence. Concentration is perfect for increasing the level of awareness. We are aware of the feelings in the body, and the mind is able, in peace, to carefully observe what is in front of him.

In addition to concentration, Buddhist meditation aims at the development of awareness, using concentration only as a tool toward that end. For example, Zen Buddhist meditation uses two separate approaches.

The first approach is the direct dive into awareness by pure force of will. The aim is to just sit down and throw everything out of your mind — everything except the pure awareness of sitting. This is very hard to achieve.

The second Zen approach is to trick the mind out of conscious thought and into pure awareness by asking a student to solve an unsolvable riddle, thus placing them in a terrible training situation. Even if Zen is helpful to a lot of people, it can be very tough.

Mindfulness with Breathing Meditation

Breath is almost the only sure thing in your life. Your breath is with you as long as you live. You can rely on it. It will always be your retreat from all your hectic surroundings.

Begin by focusing your mind on your nostrils. Start breathing in and out normally. As you breathe in, say, "breathing in..." As you breathe out, say, "breathing out..."

Your mind will typically try to go somewhere else, and often, it will do this repeatedly. Just take note of the place it went and repeat its name. Then, return your focus to your breath. It is also the same for any feelings that could arise, external distractions, etc. You just notice them, repeat in your mind what the distraction is, and gently remind yourself to return your focus to the breath.

The foundation of the teaching is complete dedication to "Anapanasati-Bhavana" (mindfulness with breathing) meditation.

The correct and complete practice of this kind of meditation is to take some truth or reality of nature and then observe, investigate, and scrutinize it in your mind with every inhalation and every exhalation.

In this type of meditation, you will contemplate the secrets of "kaya" (body), the secrets of "Vedana" (feeling), the secrets of "Citta" (mind), and the secrets of "Dhamma" (the teaching of Buddha). These four objects' secrets should be accepted into your mind and then studied.

You would start with a breath. There are many different types of breathing: long breaths, short breaths, calm breaths, violent breaths, fast breaths, and slow breaths.

You need to analyze, to examine the nature, characteristics, and functions of each kind of breath that arises. Also, you would learn how different breathing have different effects on your body.

While you are getting ready to start your meditation, first, you must choose a place that is suitable and appropriate for the practice. The site does not need to be perfect, because you cannot find such an area. Come to terms with that.

This place just needs to be quiet and peaceful, where the conditions are right and where there is the least possible disturbance. But if that is not available to you, then you can focus on your breath and be aware of other external conditions so that you can accept them. Also, whenever possible, you should choose a time of the day when there are no distractions or disturbances. But this is rarely the case, so you should just use the best time available.

There is also the consideration of the teacher. A good teacher can help, but you should not forget that no one can directly help someone else. This path is yours alone.

Next, you need to assume the appropriate sitting posture. It is essential to sit in a way that is both stable and secure, so when the mind becomes semiconscious, you will not fall over. It is also important to sit upright, with the vertebrae and spine in proper alignment, without any bends or curves. The vertebrae should sit snugly, one on top of the other, so that they fit together correctly.

At first, keep your eyes open, gazing toward the tip of your nose so that your eyes do not get involved with other distractions. If you close your eyes, you might get sleepy, so be careful about this option. Later, as you gain more experience, you will be able to meditate with your eyes closed.

You will now come to nothingness, contemplating your breath, and developing "Sati" (mindfulness or reflective awareness) by being mindful of each in-breath (inhale) and each out-breath (exhale).

Let it be natural. Do not interfere with it in any way. Then, contemplate each breath with mindfulness. How are you breathing? What is exhale like? Note your observations so you can compare them with your later experiences.

Next, find a place where you can easily observe your breath. In the beginning, take a few deep, steady breaths to find and keep this spot. It can be the tip of your nose or your lips. Once you find it, observe that point as the breath passes in and out. The breath becomes subtler and gentler as soon as you start to note it and follow it. Finally, when you stop chasing after your breath, it calms down even more. You can verify this through your own experience.

It also helps to count. You can count each inhalation as it starts, one number for each breath. If the mind wanders, start counting again. If you can count to ten without your mind wandering, good job! But you should go back to the beginning anyway.

These tricks will help you get started. When you adopt them, you will always have them at your service in your meditation and in your everyday life.

Now, when you settle into observing your breath, you can expand this a bit more.

Become aware of the three primary segments of each breath: the beginning, middle, and end.

You will feel them during the inhalation in your nose, the middle of the chest, and the abdomen, and then the reverse during exhalation. This way, you will have a better understanding of your breath, and when you master this, you can move your focus to other challenges, like your feelings and your thoughts.

Vipassana Meditation

Vipassana is the oldest of Buddhist meditation practices. It comes from the Satipatthana Sutta, which is thought to have been explained by the Buddha himself. Vipassana is a direct development of mindfulness or awareness.

When you practice vipassana meditation, your attention is gently directed to a holistic examination of the aspects of your existence. You are trained to observe more and more of the flow of your life experience.

Vipassana is very, very hard to do, even if it seems very gentle. It trains your mind to focus on attentive listening, mindful seeing, and careful testing. You will be able to "smell actually, to touch fully" and notice the changes that are taking place during these experiences.

You must learn to listen to your own thoughts without getting caught up in them. That way, you will see the truth: objects are impermanent and unsatisfactory.

Vipassana is a process of self-discovery, an active investigation in which you observe your own experiences while participating in them.

If you pursue your meditation practice with an open mind, you will succeed.

By practicing vipassana meditation, you will be able to condition yourself to see reality truly as it is. You will gain mindfulness.

Throughout your whole life, you try to make yourself feel better and happier. You desperately try to put away your fears and gain security. At the same time, your real-world experience is not affected by your wishes. When practicing vipassana meditation, you will learn to ignore your urge to live a luxurious and shallow carefree life, and you will be ready to accept reality. Then, you will be able to choose your battles wisely. Another interesting fact is that, often, real peace comes as soon as you stop chasing it.

If I can now conclude what vipassana meditation represents, I would say that it is a set of practices that opens us, step by step, to a better understanding of reality as it truly is, how things actually feel. For me, the most significant advance in my understanding of vipassana meditation is that it teaches you to stop thinking about life; instead, you just live it fully.

Vipassana will teach you to live in this moment because the past has already happened, and the future is yet to come, as Buddha said. So, make the most of this moment, and don't spoil it with endless regrets or by dreaming about a future that might never happen the way you hope it will.

Finding the Best Ways to Concentrate

It is essential to determine the best atmosphere and location for keeping your concentration at the right level to perform the task ahead.

Sometimes, you will need near-absolute silence; other times, some music will help a lot. You must find out what works for you. The best environment for others may not work for you. Even in different stages of your life, different surroundings might influence you differently. Always seek optimal conditions and try different setups.

But bear in mind that you must be able to work in less than ideal circumstances. Mindfulness meditation will help you with that immensely.

We do not need to control anything and everything. We can adapt.

You will also need to be patient. Achieving mindfulness and concentration to avoid procrastination is a process. Sometimes, it will not go as well as you would like. Be patient and persistent. Eventually, your hard work will pay off.

Live a Disciplined Life

I firmly believe that the most successful long-term cure for procrastination is to live a disciplined life. If you manage to achieve discipline in how you eat, exercise, and even meditate, you will have a much higher chance of avoiding procrastination. To have a structure in your life is very helpful.

Of course, you should not become a prisoner of those habits. Use them only when they help your cause. Stop wasting hours of your day watching YouTube, playing video games, or browsing social media.

Apart from helping you fight procrastination discipline will also help you to develop self-control and willpower.

If you are not prepared to live a disciplined life, you will struggle with procrastination. I am sure of that.

Think Concretely

Research shows that thinking in specific terms helps us stop procrastinating and start acting. When we only focus on the next step, negative thoughts and emotions get pushed into the background of our consciousness, thus helping us get started.

Simple Practices

Here are some simple hacks you can use in addition to practicing mindfulness meditation.

David Allen's 2-Minute Rule

David Allen's 2-minute rule teaches us that if a task takes less than 2 minutes to complete, you should do it immediately. Instead of filling your mind or to-do list with an endless supply of small jobs, get in the habit of getting them done the instant they appear.

After cooking or eating, wash the dishes immediately. Do not leave them in the sink for hours. The day you get the bills, pay them promptly; do not wait for "some convenient time in the future." Answer simple "yes" or "no" emails immediately instead of doing it "later." Bring out the garbage right when it's full, instead of doing it "later." Anything that takes less than two minutes do it immediately.

This will give you a small sense of accomplishment and re-train your mind to learn how to just get started and get things done, whether you feel like it or not. Those little victories go a long way in reducing procrastination.

Mel Robbins' 5-Second Rule

The 5-second rule (invented by life coach Mel Robbins) states, "If you have an impulse to act on a goal, you must physically move within 5 seconds, or your brain will kill the idea."

If you feel a sudden urge to act, you'd better get moving quickly. Don't let your mind come up with excuses. Don't let your mind force you to run away from this. Just get started immediately. Act faster. Once you get started, good things will naturally begin to follow.

Anna Black's 60-Second Timer

When you recognize the impulse to run away, hurry back into yourself instead. In the book "Mindfulness@Work," Anna Black proposes taking a stopwatch, kitchen timer, or a smartphone and set the timer to one minute. Breathe deeply for the chosen time, counting your breaths. When your 60 seconds are up, you will have an idea of how fast you are breathing.

In those moments, when you feel the desire to escape, take a mindful minute — sometimes, that's all you need to get back to neutral. When you're done, break up your goals into tiny and manageable pieces. If you manage to stay in the "now" and focus on your tasks, you will be able to accomplish your goals without feeling overwhelmed.

These rules are not substitutions for developing mindfulness. They are simple hacks to push you in the right direction. No matter what, you should stay on the path to mindfulness and a better understanding of yourself. That way, you can become less stressed-out and have much fewer reasons for procrastination. Once you can accept that you are in command of your own feelings and thoughts, you will be able to avoid procrastination in most cases. Not always.

Anyhow, a little bit of relaxing and doing things that are not important are also ways to keep your mind healthy. Just take the middle path and be moderate about it. It is crucial to integrate these three mindfulness practices into your daily habits. By learning how to tackle challenges in peaceful and fulfilling ways, you will be on your way to personal and professional success.

Do Things You Enjoy

In addition to doing all of the above, pay attention to your needs, and do things you actually enjoy. Often, procrastination is your way to vent out the building frustration caused by not being able to do the things you enjoy. If you have just been working hard for a long time and haven't done anything enjoyable lately, you are likely to lean towards meaningless activities. This can then trigger your habit of procrastinating and create more significant problems for you.

An excellent way to keep that from happening is to occasionally devote some time to your needs of enjoyment and entertainment. Make it a daily or weekly ritual to engage in some enjoyable activity, such as painting, dancing, listening to music, or doing anything else that mitigates your stress and helps you breathe. When you consistently give yourself some quality "me" time, you feel better and more content with yourself and are more able to quickly motivate yourself to complete your high-priority tasks on time.

Find Work You Love

We procrastinate on stuff we don't enjoy doing. If you can find work you truly love, procrastination will become a non-issue (concerning that work). You will feel intrinsically motivated, and you will find yourself wanting to work. Imagine you were a professional online gamer — you wouldn't procrastinate on getting up in the morning and playing, would you?

Never Give Up

When you meditate, before you can let things go, you have to skilfully allow the subconscious to rise into consciousness. All your fears, anguish, despair, and anger are allowed to become conscious.

THE PATH TO PEACE AND HAPPINESS

I n the end, we are all looking for peace and happiness. Even it seems that we want food, wealth, sex, entertainment, and respect, those are only superficial representations of a much deeper feeling of happiness.

What is happiness? It cannot be just the power to be in control of everything. Experience teaches us that you cannot control others. Instead, you can learn to control your mind, to stop being contaminated with desire and aversion.

Learn to recognize desire and not be controlled by it. You should not accept everything that happens to you. You need to have a productive relationship with your life, but with a new point of view on everyday life events. Mindfulness teaches you to change things in your life that you can, but also to accept those that you cannot.

It is crucial to be able to look carefully inside your mind, truthfully, and objectively. You must learn how to recognize those moments without judgment. Only then can you make fundamental changes in your everyday life. Let go of resistance to change, let go of your illusions and perceptions. When you achieve that, you will see yourself as you are right now. That does not mean that you need to isolate yourself from social interactions. You must fulfill your duties and obligations to your family and friends, to all fellow humans, beings, and, most importantly, to yourself.

This is your path to achieving true happiness.

Working on mindfulness, you will better understand yourself. As your understanding grows, the more compassionate you can be. You will be ready to forgive and forget and to learn to love by understanding your inner self.

This is not an issue of faith. This is an issue of confidence and experience. It is made through everyday practice and endurance on the path to discover things as they really are.

* * *

Focusing on happiness and success is the right way to achieve your goals.

This is the most important path that you must walk by yourself.

No one can do it for you. You need to be determined, be mindful, and do not give up.

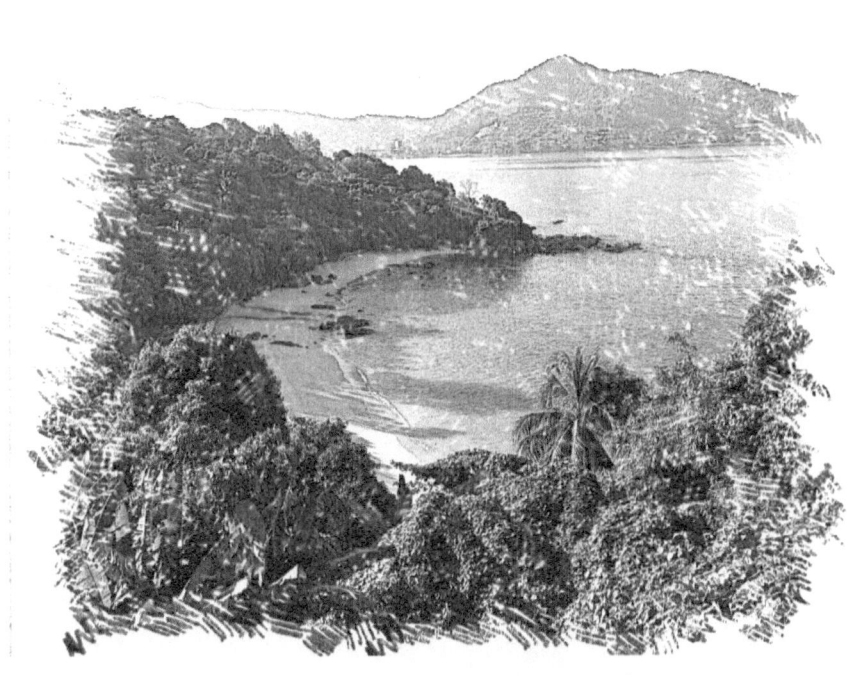

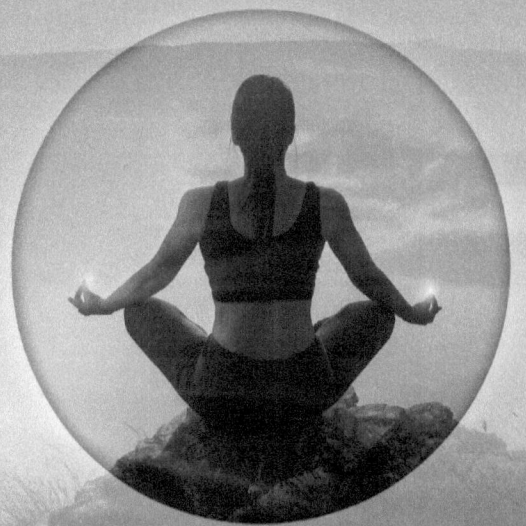

MINDFULNESS MEDITATION

A BEGINNER'S GUIDE TO YOGA MEDITATION

HOW TO RELIEVE STRESS AND FIND HAPPINESS IN YOUR LIFE

GEORGE M. POSI

BOOK 5: MINDFULNESS MEDITATION: A BEGINNER'S GUIDE TO YOGA MEDITATION

How to Relieve Stress and Find Happiness in Your Life

Table of Contents

WHAT IS MEDITATION?

I t is known from ancient times that mindfulness meditation is a powerful technique. It has been used for thousands of years to reduce anxiety, depression, stress, and help you achieve peace of mind.

Mindfulness meditation helps you train your mind to remain in the present moment, entirely calm and aware of your surroundings. Often, we become anxious and stressed because of a troubling past that we still think about or being upset about a future that is yet to come and that we have no control over. With mindfulness meditation, you will learn to live in only the present moment.

The practices of mindfulness meditation originate from Hinduism. Buddhism has adopted these techniques and improved on them, so they become integral to what is referred to as the "Buddhist path." In Buddhism, cultivating non-judgmental awareness of yourself, your feelings, and your mind is considered crucial if you want to lead a calm and peaceful life.

What is most important for the mind is to fully attend to what is taking place, to what you are doing, and to space through which you are moving. If we stop being in touch with our body and become absorbed in obsessive thoughts about stuff that has already taken place or if we always worry about the future, then we create anxiety for ourselves. Even in such moments, mindfulness is there to take us back to where we are and what we are feeling and doing.

In the yoga tradition, there is a methodology that is designed to show us the connection between every living thing. Meditation is the actual experience of this union (Advaita).

Instructions for how to meditate and description of meditation practice are found in the Yoga Sutra. This mental stillness brings the body, mind, and senses into a state of balance. This also relaxes the nervous system. Real meditation begins after we realize that our need to possess and our everlasting craving for pleasure will never be satisfied. Only then does our external pursuit turn inward, and we are in the real state of meditation. Meditation (Dhyana) in the yogic context is defined as a state of pure consciousness. When we are aware of our senses but disengaged at the same time. Our concentration allowed us to be grounded, mentally, and physically. In fact, meditation is much more than concentration. It represents an expanded state of awareness.

To achieve the state of self-realization (Samadhi), it is not enough just to focus our mind on an object apart from ourselves. We need to do more than only establish contact and get familiar with it. We need to communicate with this object and gain a deep awareness of the fact that there is no difference between this object and ourselves.

When we are separate from nature, we feel pain and suffering, according to the Yoga Sutra. To stay in contact with nature, we can make our minds stable and focused, and we can make full use of it and enable our consciousness to grow. This is best accomplished through the practice of mindfulness meditation. When you meditate, you use a technique to develop your mind, the same way you use physical exercise to build your muscles.

We all have a restless mind. Thoughts just come uninvited at any moment of the day and even at night. This is a waste of your precious mental energy, and as such, you get exhausted by these wandering thoughts. Meditation will help you to eliminate those thoughts.

How does meditation work?

The word "meditation" does not describe all Buddhist ideas embodied in the Pali word "Bhavana." It means much more and can be defined as "to develop our mental ability." Meditation is more than be willing to sit quietly and close your eyes. It is more than thinking about only the good things in your life and disregarding all that is bad. It is not about becoming overly optimistic. Meditation has everything to do with your everyday life. It is not only for monks and old people who have retired and have time for it.

In the Buddhist teachings, we learn to recognize six senses. The outside world is brought to us through the eyes, ears, nose, tongue, body, and mind. The first five are physical senses, and the mind works as a mental sense. Things you perceive through your six senses are meditation objects.

This knowledge of how to perceive the world is essential for successful meditation.

THE BENEFITS OF MEDITATION

H erbert Benson, MD, a researcher at Harvard University Medical School, found that relaxation is not the goal of meditation, but that it is often a result. The relaxation response, as he called it, is "an opposite, involuntary response that causes a reduction in the activity of the sympathetic nervous system."

Various studies on the relaxation response have also found the benefits of reducing activity in the nervous system:

- Lower blood pressure
- Improved blood circulation
- Lower heart rate
- Less perspiration
- Slower respiratory rate
- Less anxiety
- Lower blood cortisol levels
- More feelings of satisfied well-being
- Less stress
- Deeper relaxation

Those are mainly short-term benefits, but some researchers suspect that there are some long-term benefits as well. But remember that the purpose of meditation is not to achieve any benefits from it. Be present in this moment and at this place is the ultimate goal of meditation.

According to Buddhist teachings, the mind being free from attachment is the ultimate benefit of meditation. Letting go of things our mind cannot control and maintaining the sense of inner harmony are the keys to the path of achieving true liberation. Our mind will learn how to stop needlessly following desires or clinging to experiences and thus become genuinely calm.

Research has confirmed that profound psychological and physiological changes happen when we meditate. Meditation changes specific processes in the brain and other involuntary processes of the body.

Meditation helps you to manage stress. Reducing stress improves your overall physical health and emotional well-being. Meditation raises the quality of your life by teaching you to be fully alert, aware, and alive. In fact, we are not meditating to gain something. We meditate to let go of things that we don't need.

TYPES OF MEDITATION

T here are many different types of meditation. You should try some of them and decide which is your favorite, which one works the best for you. Do your research and tests, but do not give up easily. For you to know if this is the right technique for you, you must let it settle, let it become a part of your routine. If you are not satisfied with the feelings provided by this type of meditative practice after a few weeks, try something different.

Here are some of the main types of meditative practices, but remember that there are a lot of variations on all of them.

Mindfulness with Breathing Meditation

In this type of meditation, you will start with a breath. You will learn how different types of breathing have different effects on your body. We will explain the posture and place for meditation. Let me just tell you that the site for your meditation practice does not need to be perfect because you cannot find such an area. No place is perfect.

It is important to sit in a way that is both stable and secure, so when the mind becomes semiconscious, you will not fall over. It is also important to sit upright, with the vertebrae and spine in proper alignment, without any bends or curves. The vertebrae should sit snugly, one on top of the other, so that they fit together correctly.

At first, keep your eyes open, gazing toward the tip of your nose so that your eyes do not get involved with other distractions. If you close your eyes, you might get sleepy, so be careful about this option. Later, as you gain more experience, you will be able to meditate even with your eyes closed—without falling asleep.

Let your breath be natural. Do not interfere with it in any way. Then, contemplate each breath with mindfulness. How are you breathing? What is exhale like? Note your observations so you can compare them with your later experiences.

It also helps to count. You can count each inhalation as it starts, one number for each breath. If your mind wanders, start counting again. If you can count to ten without the mind wandering, go back to the count of "one" anyway.

These tricks will help you get started. When you adopt them, you will always have them at your service in your meditation and in your everyday life.

Metta Meditation

As a part of your meditation routine, you can focus your inner attention on someone you know who might benefit from an extra dose of kindness and care. Send this person love, happiness, and well-being. In the Buddhist tradition, this is called Metta meditation practice, and it can benefit you greatly.

"Metta" can be translated from Pali (the language of Buddha) as "loving-kindness" or "friendly love." Many Buddhists regard this type of meditation as the default kind. Metta meditation is constructed of four components: Metta, Karuna (compassion), Mudita (sympathetic joy), and Upekkha (balanced mind).

Metta represents the desire to see peace and success in your life, as well as to be free from harm. This then extends to members of your family and friends, and later, it becomes universal.

For Metta meditation to be successful, you must have engaged in putting forth the right effort. You must really mean the words that you are saying to yourself while meditating. Developing Metta —developing loving-kindness toward yourself— is, therefore, crucial in overcoming frustration within oneself. This gradual reduction of frustration is the first benefit that one earns from Metta meditation.

In the beginning, choose yourself as the meditation object. Repeat to yourself in your thoughts, "May I be free from (state first negative condition). May I be free from (other negative condition). May I be able to (state first positive condition). May I be able to (other negative condition)." Repeat these two to five times.

You will next dedicate your thoughts to people you care about: your parents, children, spouse, or siblings. Visualize them and repeat: "May they be free from (say your choice of one negative condition). May they be free from (say your choice of a second negative condition). May they be able to (say your choice of a positive condition). May they be able to (say your choice of a second positive condition)." You can wish them to be free from illness, and to have good health, or some more specific condition that you know is appropriate for them.

In this way, you will develop mindfulness of your feelings of well-being, your desire to be free from harm, and suffering, and this then leads to the development of Metta for yourself and the people closest to you.

Now, you choose a neutral person. They may be someone from work or someone you have come across anywhere you've gone, someone you neither like nor dislike. This person is entirely neutral. Direct your Metta thoughts to that person in the same way as you did before.

In your first Metta meditations, do not use the people you have been in conflict with or had arguments with. Do not start with people of the gender you're attracted to, as this can provoke lust. Also, do not use those who have died, for this can stir up sorrow.

You can also have the next part of Metta meditation directed to an unspecified person (your whole country, world, any other living being, etc.). You can try doing this in your next meditations.

Vipassana Meditation

The purpose of meditation is to clear your mind and get rid of greed, hatred, and jealousy. Meditation helps you to bring your mind to a state of concentration, insight, and tranquility, and by doing so, you can achieve awareness.

You might like to practice Vipassana meditation to help you face reality or to experience life just as it is. After that, you can change the way you live.

You must learn to listen to your own thoughts without getting caught up in them. That way, you will see the truth: objects are impermanent and unsatisfactory.

By practicing Vipassana meditation, you will be able to condition yourself to see reality truly as it is. You will gain mindfulness.

There is no unique technique to it. You are practicing Vipassana when you focus on breathing—just letting any emotions, feelings, and thoughts to arise. You acknowledge them, accept them, and then let them go. You just need to sit and genuinely commit to doing Vipassana meditation.

Other Forms of Meditation

Within the Judeo-Christian tradition, there are two leading practices: prayer and contemplation. Prayer can be described as an address to God.

Contemplation is a process of conscious thought about a specific topic, like a religious ideal or religious script. Prayer and reflection are exercises in concentration.

Hindu tradition treats yogic meditation as purely concentrative. It focuses the mind on a single object, not allowing it to wander. In advanced practice, yogis proceed to expand it by assuming more complex objects of meditation.

In addition to concentration, Buddhist meditation aims toward the development of awareness, using concentration only as a tool toward that end. The aim of Zen Buddhist meditation is to just sit down and throw everything out of your mind. You keep only the pure awareness of sitting. This is very hard to achieve.

On the other side of "toughness" is Tantric Buddhism. So, there are many ways to achieve peace of mind.

MEDITATION IN MOTION

While I was at a Suan Mokkh meditation retreat in Chaiya, Thailand, I had the opportunity to try different types of meditative practice (like yoga, Taiji, or Qigong). This group that I particularly like can be called "meditation in motion." Every morning, we had one of these practices, and I must say that I feel that by beginning the day in mindful motion, your whole day starts developing in a much more positive fashion.

Taiji (Tai Chi)

Taiji (tai chi), is a Chinese martial art practiced not only for its physical but also for its health benefits and meditation practices. It is another excellent example of the meditation-in-motion concept. In its movement, Taiji practice embodies the philosophy of yin and yang.

In the latest period, Taiji has developed worldwide recognition, with the focus on improving personal physical and mental health.

Focusing your mind on the movements helps you achieve calm and clarity of the mind. Again, according to Wikipedia, it is "considered to teach the use of leverage through the joints based on coordination and relaxation, rather than muscular tension, to neutralize, yield, or initiate attacks. The slow, repetitive work involved in the process of learning how that leverage is generated gently and [how it] measurably increases, as well as opens, the internal circulation (breath, body heat, blood, lymph, peristalsis)."

One may say that Taiji is both health training and meditation practice, along with its original martial art component.

Qigong

"Qigong" is pronounced "Chi-Gung."

"Qigong is a holistic system of coordinated body posture and movement, breathing, and meditation used for the purposes of health, spirituality, and martial arts training. With roots in Chinese medicine, philosophy, and martial arts, Qigong is traditionally viewed by the Chinese and throughout Asia as a practice to cultivate and balance qi (pronounced approximately as "chi"), translated as "life energy" (Wikipedia).

Deep rhythmic breathing, slow-flowing movement, and a calm meditative state of mind are the focuses of Qigong practice and philosophy.

The core of Qigong contains practices that coordinate body, breath, and mind. It has its origins in Chinese philosophy. Qigong practice consists of both moving and still meditation in various postures, massage, and chanting, etc. As it is primarily a form of moving meditation, Qigong practice involves carefully choreographed movement, coordinated with breath and awareness.

Yoga

For thousands of years, yoga has been one of the most effective ways to manage stress, gain happiness, and establish peace of mind. It can also help to reduce body pain, as well as increase flexibility and body strength.

In Sanskrit, the word "yoga" is usually used to signify connection or union. Yoga is actually the whole process of being more aware of who you are.

The origin of yoga can be traced back to more than 5,000 years ago in northern India. In the oldest sacred texts known as the Rig Veda, we find the first reference to the word "yoga." This text contained mantras, rituals, and songs used by the Vedic priests (Brahmans).

In a broad sense, yoga represents a group of physical, mental, and spiritual practices. In the Western world, it is often simplified to assume physical exercise postures (asanas), mainly referring to Hatha yoga. Even though texts about Hatha yoga date from between the 9th and 11th centuries, with origins in tantra, it is only in the 19th and 20th centuries that yoga became known to Westerners.

As stated on Wikipedia, "Yoga as exercise is a physical activity consisting largely of asanas, often connected by flowing sequences called Vinyasas, sometimes accompanied by the breathing exercises of Pranayama, and usually ending with a period of relaxation or meditation."

It is often forgotten that the goals of yoga are spiritual liberation, achieving inner peace, and being in harmony with nature. Meditation is a spiritual part of yoga that cannot be set apart. That why we sometimes refer to yoga practice as "meditation in motion."

The Connection Between Yoga and Meditation

In today's hectic world, we look for activities that help us calm our minds. We know from our experience that techniques to calm your mind can help fight anxiety and improve our mood. We call those activities "mindfulness."

It is accepted that not only does yoga help to fight depression, but it also improves your physical well-being. Regular practice lightens your mood and takes you away from your everyday troubles, even if just for that moment when we practice. A combination of physical and mental incentives that yoga offers should be embraced and broadened by regular practice. It will help you to manage stress effectively.

Yoga also helps your sense of accomplishment after you finish your daily yoga routine. It also prepares you to enter deeper states of mind by practicing breathing (Pranayama) and performing different meditative methods inside your yoga practice. Yoga postures are intended to prepare your body for meditation.

When we begin to slow our breath and begin to sync it with our movement, we become calm. Then, we grow closer to the single-minded purpose. By slowing down, we begin to accomplish more, and we keep our attention in the present moment. Yoga not only helps to strengthen our body, but raises our awareness, and prepares us for meditation. Proper breathing helps calm your mind. It gives a rhythm to your thoughts and helps create a peaceful structure of the mind.

Meditation and yoga are interrelated. Yogis say, "Where the breath flows, the mind goes." Yoga, like meditative chanting, can allow the energy to flow upward and to open our heart to the higher chakras and higher consciousness.

Shavasana, the Yoga Meditation for Relaxation

The most popular pose in yoga for meditation practice is Shavasana (corpse pose). It is practically the most integral part of any yoga class. Though yoga is often described as "Moving Meditation," this pose requires you to be completely calm and still, thus entering a meditative state.

The word "Shavasana" has Sanskrit origins. We practice the Shavasana pose by lying face-up on the ground, arms and legs comfortably spread, and with eyes closed. To begin, we will gradually scan our body down from head to toe, relaxing one body part at a time. Keep awareness of the parts of the body that feel relaxed. Notice which parts are still tense.

Do you feel comfortable or uncomfortable? Is your body light or heavy? If thoughts arise, just notice them and let your breath carry them away. Let your breath bring you to the place of stillness. The more you practice, the easier it gets to achieve this. In time, your breathing will become quieter, slower, and more profound. You will become really calm, not only when practicing but in your everyday life as well.

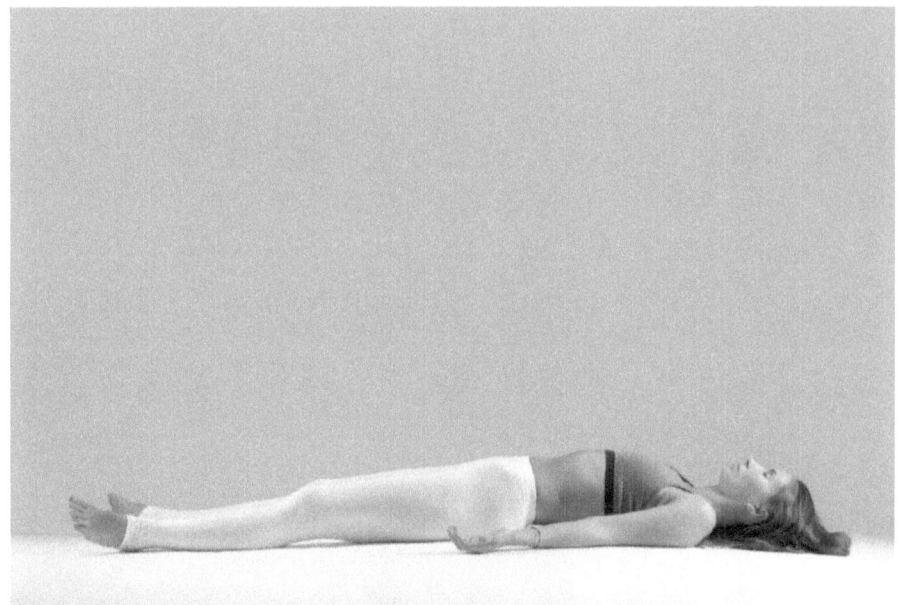

Corpse pose (Shavasana)

Many beginners thought that Shavasana pose is easy, but more experienced yoga students know that Shavasana can actually be the most challenging and beneficial of all the poses. That's because the essence of Shavasana is to relax the mind and body while remaining present and maintaining awareness.

Shavasana helps you relax, causing a lowered heart rate, a sense of calm, and a decreased release of stress hormones, like adrenaline and cortisol. It makes us feel good. And that was just what we wanted. Now we can approach everyday problems and challenges and solve them using our calm mind.

MEDITATION PRACTICE

I n order to have a successful meditation practice, you need regular, daily exercise, choose to just sit quietly and watch what happens. For that time, ignore your phone, don't answer the doorbell, don't add another item to your to-do list in your mind. Just sit and observe your thoughts as they come and pass through your mind. You will find it very hard, if not impossible, to have even half a minute of having a calm mind. It is only possible if you are determined and committed.

It is best to simply add it to the end of your daily yoga exercises, your asana practice. You can choose to practice meditation in some other part of the day, but the important thing is that you find a time that works best for you. Be patient; do not rush your practice. Soon, you will be able to have longer and longer sessions, and you will feel real benefits. To start, even 5 to 10 minutes is enough. You will probably be surprised by how difficult it is to sit quietly for "only" 10 minutes. Later, try to lengthen your meditation practice by 5 minutes every week until you reach your desired length. It can be anything from 20 to 60 minutes a day—or more if you can spare the time.

Almost all people that practice yoga also practices some form of meditation. Often, it is just a part of their yoga practice, but also as a separate practice for achieving their peace of mind. So over time, practitioners of yoga tend to seek some more complex meditation practices and to go deeper into the philosophy behind the techniques of meditation.

When and Where to Practice

Try to meditate at the same time and in the same place every day. This place should be quiet, a place where you will not be disturbed. If this is not available to you, it is essential to have in mind that you can meditate in other circumstances. It is not a reason to quit.

Some people are the most relaxed and ready to meditate in the morning. It helps them start the day with a positive mind. Evening meditation is more suitable for others because it calms their mind before sleeping at night.

Meditation Postures

Sitting on the floor is the most common meditation posture. You can also do walking or standing meditation. The only essential things are maintaining proper position and staying focused for the entire time.

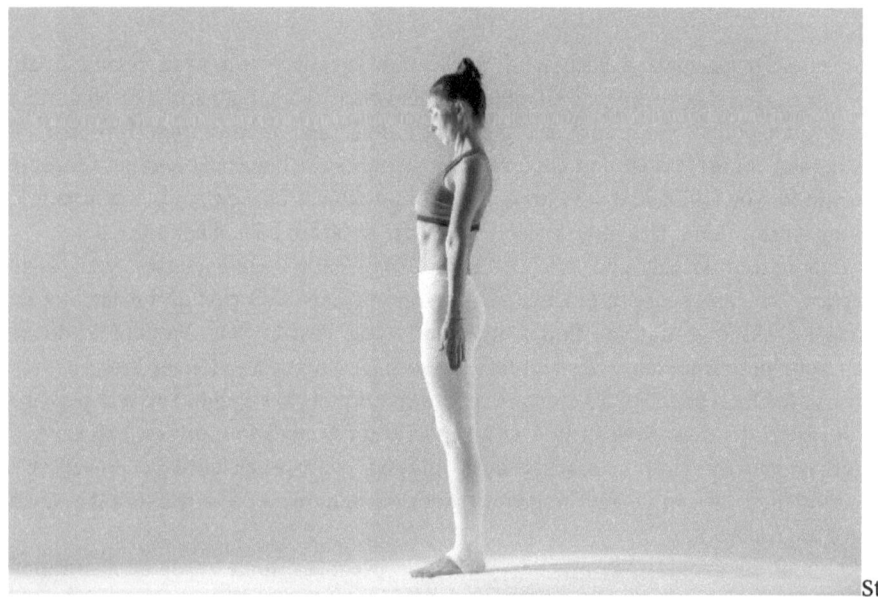

Standing pose (Tadasana)

Standing

Standing is another meditation practice that you can use in combination with sitting meditation, to rest your body. It can be used as a complete practice in case you want to additionally build physical, mental, and spiritual strength. Stand with your feet about a hip's distance apart. Don't lock your knees, and let your arms rest comfortably at your sides. Your shoulders should be pulled back and down, chest open, neck long, head floating on top, and chin parallel to the floor. You can keep your eyes opened or closed.

Walking

It is one of the most widely used postures. You should walk slowly and consciously and focus on each step. Let your arms move freely at your sides. Your breath should be in synchronization with your footsteps.

Choose a quiet place. Focus on the individual parts of your steps: how you lift your foot, how you move it forward, how you put it back on the ground. Your pace should be moderate, and you should have enough space to make about 15 to 30 steps in one line. Then, you stop and turn. It is essential to make every move consciously, contemplating the movement in your mind. This involvement in your steps is your meditation practice. Often, practitioners combine walking and sitting meditation in successive sessions, sitting down for 30 minutes, then walking for 30 minutes, and so on.

Sitting

You can meditate while sitting on the floor or on a chair—whichever works for you. It is important to keep the spine upright, and the body relaxed. If you are sitting on the floor, in the beginning, you can assume for the basic Cross-Legged Pose (Sukhasana). If you are very flexible, you can sit down in Lotus Pose (Padmasana). You can also sit and kneel on a small, slanted wooden bench. Place your hands comfortably on your lap, knees, or thighs. Your palms can be up or down.

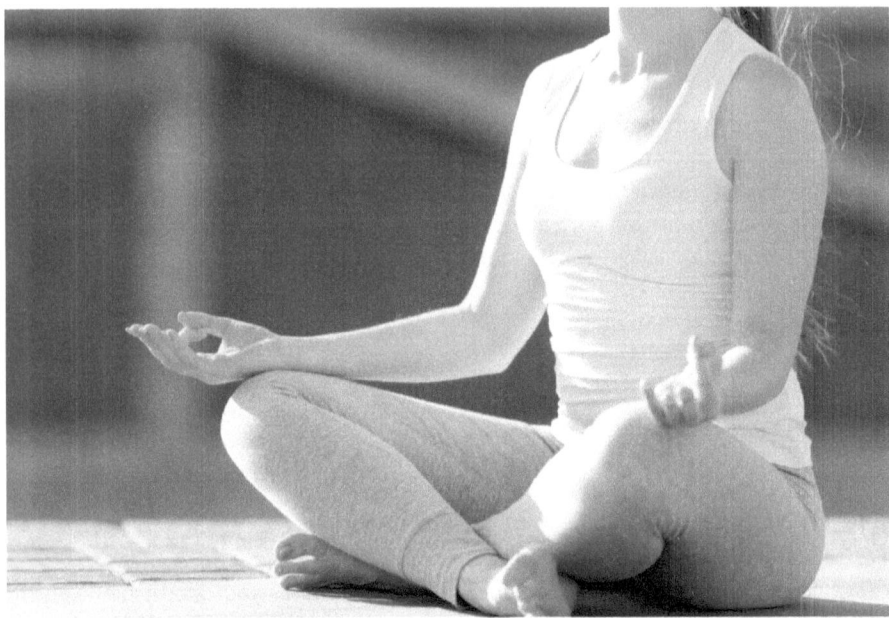

Cross-Legged Pose (Sukhasana)

Lying Down

It is also common to finish your yoga practice with lying-down meditation (Shavasana). In that case, be sure to assume a comfortable position and have the appropriate support under your head and knees if needed. Lie down on your back with your arms at your sides, palms facing upward. Your body needs to be fully relaxed. Your eyes can be open or closed, depending on if you feel you might fall asleep. It is a less physically challenging pose, but it requires more mental strength to remain awake and focused.

Methods of Meditation

The most common method of meditation is focusing on your breath. It is very convenient because it is always there for us. In the Buddhist tradition, this is the standard method of meditation. It is the simple observation of your breath as you inhale and exhale. In the beginning, you can count your inhalations and exhalations, and later, you will get accustomed to just observing various sensations that your breathing produces. In other teachings and traditions, there are additional methods and styles of meditation. In advanced stages, you will be able to observe your whole body and how it reacts to every breath you take.

Observing physical sensations is another way to meditate. You should do the same as you would when concentrating on your breaths. You can follow the sweat on your palms, the weight of your body pressing against the floor, the back pain from sitting for too long... You can also observe your emotions. Stick to your focus for the whole meditation practice. This method of meditation practice is more challenging than focusing on your breath, so it is not recommended for complete beginners. As a beginner, you can instead use mantras and visualizations together with concentrating on your breathing. In the end, you will need to find for yourself what helps develop the calmness of your mind the most.

Mantra, or silently or audibly repeating a word or phrase, is another ubiquitous method of meditation. You must choose a word or phrase that is calming to you, such as "peace," "love," or "joy."

You can use affirmations as well when you breathe out. If you repeat to yourself a phrase like "I feel relaxed, I feel peaceful," then you can calm your mind and meditate. Other options include using a recording of chants or listening to relaxing music.

You can also do visualizations, or you could imagine your favorite spot in nature with your eyes closed. You can direct your gaze toward an object in front of you. You can even possibly choose a lit candle, a flower, or a picture of a deity.

Once you find what works for you, you'll want to maintain that practice indefinitely, but in the beginning, try to give various methods a chance for some time, like one month, to be sure what is best for you.

Your thoughts will wander. It happens to most experienced meditators, so this should not discourage you. You will, in that case, just gently remind yourself to go back to your object of meditation and start over. It will happen again and again. This is also how you improve your focus and willpower.

BECOMING PEACEFUL WITH YOUR THOUGHTS

Find your own meditation style.

It is not easy to have an empty mind. This is true not only for beginners but also for everyone who has really tried to achieve this goal. In this book, we have some tools that can help you get started, like with guided meditation practice, books, or friends that are already practicing meditation. It is usual to start by focusing on your breath and then gain focus. In the later stages of your practice, you can experiment with other types of meditation and find out which ones work for you. Usually, people combine a few different types of meditation practice, depending on how they feel that day.

Get rid of distractions.

Be sure to find a quiet place, but if one is not available to you, do not worry. You can create your own quiet place in time, in your mind. Turn off your mobile phone, forget about things that happened yesterday, and, most importantly, do not think about what you must do today. Do not let distractions defeat you. It is not easy, but in time, it will get more and more manageable. Assume the posture of your choice and then allow your breath and energy to flow freely.

Establish a habit.

Try to meditate regularly at the same time and place every day. But this is not a must. Just remember to practice every day, making it a habit, almost like you brush your teeth or take a morning shower. You will find, in time, that your mind will ask for your daily meditation practice itself.

Be patient.

Success will not come overnight; it never does. Almost every experienced meditator will say to you that establishing a practice is merely showing up every day. This is not entirely true. You need to put some effort into your practice and have patience. It may take months before you can really feel some progress. If you are genuinely committed to meditation practice, then the results will eventually show themselves. Do not quit.

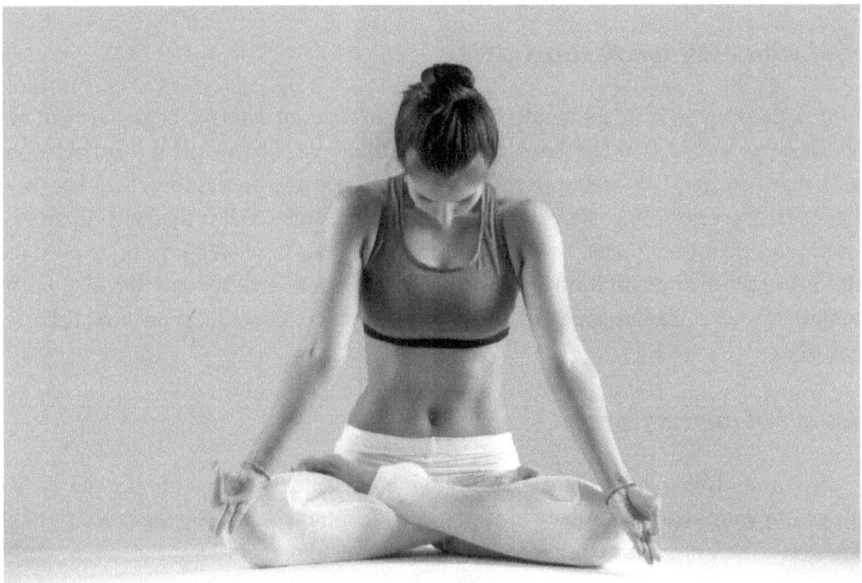

Lotus Pose (Padmasana)

Find the joy.

I think the most important thing is to find joy in meditation. We are all doing this because we want to feel better. We want to feel peace of mind, happiness, and joy. Without this, it really isn't worth it. Give it a chance to become your true nature and to sink deeply into your everyday life. Have an open mind. You will find how small, daily wins contribute so much to your whole mental health. You will see how small losses are not worth stressing out about. Let go of toxic people and look at dark situations with optimism. Your life will become much better. You will start to feel joy.

Just start meditating.

The first step can be the hardest. If you have trouble finding the right time, right place, or right mood to start, maybe it would be better to join a group or class. Later, you can broaden this practice with some guided video meditations, or you could just try to sit alone again. Make this first step into a mindfulness practice. Give it a fair chance.

Challenges You May Face

When you start your practice, and even before that, you may face some of your fears or worries. Some people are afraid to be alone with their own thoughts. It is possible that, during meditation, some thoughts that you were trying to avoid will emerge. But the purpose of mindfulness meditation is actually to train your mind to recognize them as bad habits and how to learn to let them go.

There is no point in dwelling in the past. You cannot change it.

You can learn from your past, of course. Just do not let the past become the source of your stress today. The same applies to the fear of an uncertain future. It may never come. Do plan and prepare for the future, but do not let it preoccupy your mind. This fear can be replaced by full mindfulness that anchors you in the present.

Your mind always wanders around. It cannot stand still, but this is not a reason to worry. Everybody's mind does just that. The way to calm your mind is to let go of preconceived notions and expectations. Don't expect to instantly feel better or to solve all your troubles. Just dedicate the next 5 to 20 minutes to meditation. During meditation, as good or bad feelings arise, let go of them. They are just distractors from the present moment. Your goal is to stay neutral and objective. When those thoughts occur, just gently steer your focus to the breath or the object of meditation in your practice. Do that as many times as needed. In time, you will need to do this less and less, and you will start to feel all the benefits of your meditation practice.

Is It Working for You?

You mustn't have any expectations for your meditation practice. The goal is to be in the moment and to let go of your regrets about the past or your expectations for the future. Also, we are not used to sitting on the floor for a long time. We might get uncomfortable or even feel some pain. You can change the position in that case, but try to make that choice consciously with intention and to not do it too often. Meditation shouldn't cause you to feel stressed or physically uncomfortable. Try to relax, but if you still feel uncomfortable, you can reduce the length of your meditation. You can even change your position from sitting to standing, for example.

There is also the consideration of a teacher. A good teacher can help, but you should not forget that no one can directly help someone else.

Personally, I find that I have better meditation practice when in a group. Try to join a community of yogis or meditators. There are many groups with different meditation techniques, even goals, so there is a wide range of choices for you. You may find that meditation retreats work for you. I find them enlightening. Do not quit easily, and be patient and consistent. You will probably find the results to be lifechanging.

YOU NEED TO PRACTICE EVERY DAY

T here are many ways to achieve your peace of mind. Meditation is one of the most helpful tools for doing just that. It does not matter which technique or method you choose. It is important to be persistent in your practice and patient when expecting the results. You really must practice (almost) every day to be able to have some effects. It can be hard at the beginning, but once you develop the habit, it gets much more comfortable, and it becomes part of who you are.

The present moment is the only place and time where you can decide what your answer will be to what life puts before you. The past is irreversibly behind you; there is no more than that, except for the memories in your mind and this very moment. The future doesn't exist either, except as thoughts in the present moment. So, all that exists is only now created through a mixture of causes and conditions, most of which you cannot control. The one and only choice that is under your control is your reaction here and now.

When you notice that your mind begins to preoccupy you with thoughts of the future or the past, gently restore it to the present moment by looking closely at the sky or the people around you.

Even though the reward is valuable, it is a big challenge as well. Thus, it is necessary to arm yourself with patience.

CONCLUSION

T hank you again for reading this book! I hope this book was able to help you to learn how to improve your mental health through the practice of mindfulness meditation, to create your inner peace, and to make your life better.

If you like this book, please follow me on:
Facebook https://www.facebook.com/gmposi/
Twitter https://twitter.com/george_posi
Instagram https://www.instagram.com/georgemposi
YouTube https://www.youtube.com/channel/UCmffykN4Iq8TY_1yyUWdoeA

Share how did you like my work on Facebook or Twitter with your friends!
Visit my blog site https://georgemposi.com

Finally, if you enjoyed this book, would you be kind enough to leave an honest review for it on Amazon.

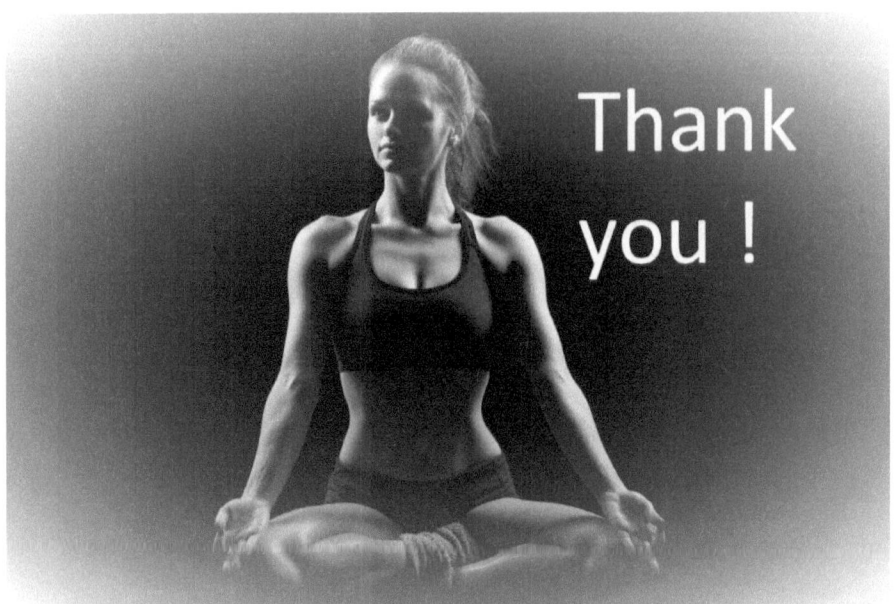

* Image Designed by Yanalya / Freepik

ABOUT THE AUTHOR

George M. Posi is an internet author and publisher and experienced entrepreneur. For the past 30 years, he has been the owner and manager of his own IT company. Five years ago, he started his journey towards mindfulness and began to seek new challenges. Then he promised himself that all business that he does must be done with respect and kindness to himself and to others.

George M. Posi started writing and publishing books as a way to reach as many people he can, to help others commit to this value in every area of their lives through self-development, including health, fitness, emotions, mindset, and spirituality.

He is grateful for all the experiences that he had in his life this first 55 years. All of those, positive and negative, helped him learn valuable life lessons. His life has since truly changed. His mission is to give back and serve others and to be a positive example of the unlimited possibilities that life offers for those that are genuinely committed to seeking mindfulness in their everyday activities.

Visit the website https://georgemposi.com, as well as YouTube channel Mindfulness Journey, where he openly and passionately shares all his experiences that have made a measurable difference to the quality of his life and will for yours as well.

Topics that George M. Posi writes about are Health and Fitness, Yoga, Mind and Beliefs, Emotions, Mission and Purpose, Productivity, Spirituality, and more...

www.ingramcontent.com/pod-product-compliance
Lightning Source LLC
Chambersburg PA
CBHW030633220526

45463CB00004B/1506